PERFUME

THE ULTIMATE
GUIDE TO THE WORLD'S
FINEST FRAGRANCES

BY NIGEL GROOM

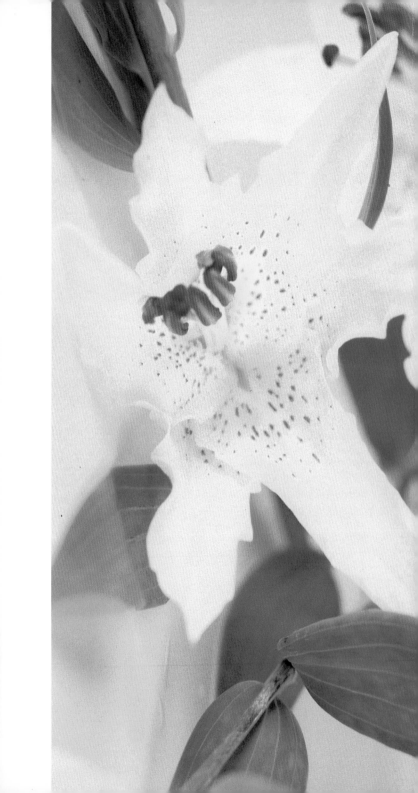

PERFUME

THE ULTIMATE
GUIDE TO THE WORLD'S
FINEST FRAGRANCES

BY NIGEL GROOM

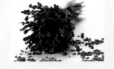

RUNNING PRESS
PHILADELPHIA · LONDON

Dedication
To Lorna, with love

A QUINTET BOOK

Copyright © 1999 Quintet Publishing Limited

All rights reserved under the Pan American and International Copyright Conventions. First
Published in the United States of America in 1999 by Running Press Book Publishers.

*This book may not be reproduced in whole or in part in any form or by any means, electronic or
mechanical, including photocopying, recording or by an information storage or retrieval system now
known or hereafter invented, without written permission from the Publisher and copyright holder.*

9 8 7 6 5 4 3 2 1
Digit on the right indicates number of this printing

ISBN 0-7624-0606-2

Library of Congress
Cataloguing-in-Publication Number
LOC 99-70310

This book was designed and produced by
Quintet Publishing Limited
6 Blundell Street
London N7 9BH

CREATIVE DIRECTOR: **richard dewing**
ART DIRECTOR: **paula marchant**
DESIGN: **balley design associates**
DESIGNERS: **simon balley and joanna hill**
SENIOR EDITOR: **clare hubbard**
EDITOR: **andrew armitage**
PHOTOGRAPHER: **tim ferguson hill**

Typeset in Great Britain by Central Southern Typesetters, Eastbourne
Manufactured in Hong Kong by Regent Publishing Services Ltd
Printed in China by Leefung-Asco Printers Ltd

This book may be ordered by mail from the publisher.
Please add $2.50 for postage and handling.
But try your bookstore first!

Running Press
Book Publishers
125 South Twenty-second Street
Philadelphia, Pennsylvania 19103–4399

Visit us on the web!
www.runningpress.com

contents

INTRODUCTION

O nly now are we beginning to understand the complexity of the mechanism by which we smell. However, what we do know is how much fragrance can affect our sense of well-being, influence our feelings toward one another, and in particular, awaken our memories of the past. Sight and sound can move the emotions, particularly through art and music, in a way that is not hard to comprehend, but smell, in particular that agreeable part of it which we call perfume, operates in a strangely mysterious way. Kipling wrote, "Scents are surer than sounds or sights to make your heartstrings crack." The perfumer, with his extraordinary ability to control fragrant material, can use this fact to create mood, romance, glamour, nostalgia, and sheer pleasure.

This book tells the story of perfume—from the temples of ancient lands to the glamour industry that it is today, where there is a perfume to suit every image, every mood, and every occasion. This is followed by a directory of select perfume houses which should give you a better understanding of the range of fragrances available so that you can select the scent to suit your own personality, your own sense of style. It will also, I hope, provide you with new enthusiasm for this absorbing and fascinating subject.

NIGEL GROOM

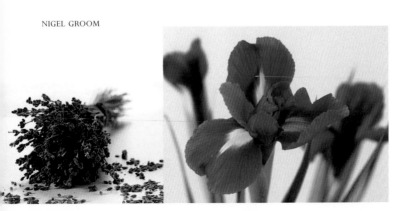

the STORY
of PERFUME

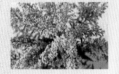

THE DEVELOPMENT
OF AN INDUSTRY

W e can say with conviction that perfume is as old as humanity, for there were surely herbs and flowers with beautiful scents long before human beings arrived on the worldly scene. But our knowledge of the earliest history of the use of perfume is vague and and has recently become even more so.

Perfume historians, working through time, felt they had reached firm ground with the series of murals in Queen Hatshepsut's temple in Thebes, which show an Egyptian fleet sailing off to fetch myrrh and other exotic aromatics from the Land of Punt 3,500 years ago. Myrrh and frankincense, staples of ancient perfume, grew only in south Arabia and Somalia, so somewhere there, after sailing down the Red Sea, lay Punt. Or so it always seemed.

Now it has been convincingly shown that the Egyptian ships journeyed up the River Nile, going further than ever previously believed possible and finding the land of Punt on the shores of Lake Albert, in Uganda. But frankincense and myrrh do not grow in that region, so we are back into uncertainty. Perhaps it is just as well. Perfume has always thrived on a little mystery and mystique.

In those very early days incense was as important as fragrant oils. Our very word *perfume* is Latin for "through smoke." Incense wafted prayers to the gods in heaven as much as it pleased the olfactory nerves and concealed bad drains. The famous *kyphi* incense, a heavy concoction, was burned in the temples at every sunset as well as in the homes at night.

BELOW: *Perfume cones drip fragrance onto the heads of women in ancient Egypt.*

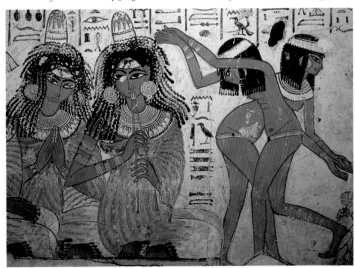

The Greeks and Romans

The Egyptians made perfumes and unguents too, steeping fragrant plants in oil and wringing out the liquid through a cloth, or soaking flower petals into fat which absorbed and preserved their fragrance.

The ancient Greeks, whose perfumers were women, enlarged and improved their Egyptian inheritance, and by Roman times vast quantities of myrrh and frankincense imported from Arabia were being supplemented with magical new ingredients collected by sea from India.

The richer Romans indulged to excess. Floors and walls were sprinkled with perfume, pet horses and dogs rubbed with it, the standards of victorious armies sprayed with it. Rose petals were scattered in abundance. But the Empire, like the perfumes, did not last.

The Arabs and Europe

A major step in the history of perfume occurred in the early Middle Ages, when the Arabs developed a technique for the large-scale distillation of plants. Huge areas of Persia were put to growing roses for rose oil and Baghdad of the Arabian Nights tales became a city of fragrances. Powerful new scent materials were found, too, like musk, which was even mixed into the mortar used to build new mosques and palaces to make them scented.

For centuries perfumery was an Arab art, almost forgotten in northern Europe. Then Crusaders began to return from the Levant with wonderfully fragrant concoctions in their luggage—gifts for wives and girlfriends—and a new demand was stimulated.

The first stage of European perfumery really began in the

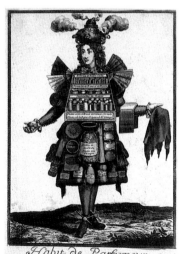

ABOVE: *Ancient Roman perfume burner.*
RIGHT: *The Perfumer's Dress, a seventeenth century engraving by Engelbrecht.*

Habit de Parfumeur

sixteenth century when Catherine de Medici, coming from Italy to marry the future king, made perfume the fashionable thing in Paris. Suddenly everybody wanted gloves of perfumed leather. The best place to get them from was Grasse, which was to thrive on this trade and develop its fragrance industry so effectively that it was soon the perfume capital of the world.

Right into Victorian times the basis of perfumery had changed little from the days of Queen Elizabeth I of England. Techniques were improved, of course, and the "juice," as perfumers now name their product, became more sophisticated, better lasting, finer scented. But then the industrial age arrived

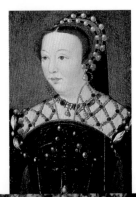

and the middle classes, suddenly much richer, found perfume being produced on an industrial scale which they too could now afford. The change was made possible by the development of synthetics. With them splendid fragrances could be produced on a large scale. But perfumers had to learn a lot more about chemistry in order to do this.

LEFT: *Catherine de Medici made perfume fashionable in Europe.*
BELOW: *Elizabeth Hurley—the "face" of Estée Lauder.*

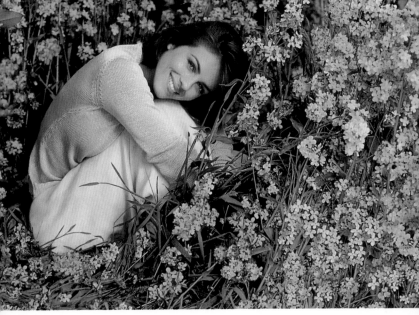

Fragrance and Fashion

Once clothes began to be mass-produced, fashion gave perfumery another huge fillip. As the couturier Paul Poiret was the first to understand, a well-dressed woman was a fragrant one, perfume adding to her glamour. Jean Patou echoed this; to him perfume was "one of the most important accessories of a woman's dress." At first couturiers such as Worth would give their clients little bottles of perfume as gifts; then, like Lanvin, they began to sell them within the store. Soon they found they could make more money from the perfumes than from the dresses.

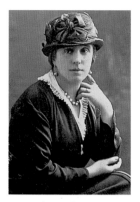

ABOVE: *Jeanne Lanvin—one of the first women to open a perfume house.*

Nowadays, a dress designer will add glamour to his or her reputation by issuing a profitable signature perfume, while the couture of famous firms like Dior, Givenchy, or Yves St Laurent may be completely subsidized by their revenues from successful fragrances.

Perfume does not, of course, sell itself, and a huge industry has built up around the processes of marketing it. First and foremost it must have an attractive bottle. But the packaging too can greatly influence sales and there are now large companies that specialize in providing this.

Advertising has always been important, as the high artistry of early advertisements reveals. The press and television are now used lavishly and in a major launch several million "scent strips" with samples of the fragrance may be placed in magazines. Extra glamour is often introduced by using a famous model or film star as the face to be associated with the perfume—like Kate Moss with Obsession or Elizabeth Hurley with Estée Lauder Pleasures.

Launching one perfume into the worldwide market nowadays can cost several million dollars. But the rewards of success make that well worthwhile. If it is a real success it may become a classic, an overused word these days which ought really to be reserved as an accolade for a perfume that has defied fashion changes and lasted on the market for at least a generation. If you can still buy the perfume your mother used when she was a girl, you can be assured that it will be a very good perfume indeed.

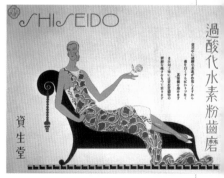

ABOVE: *Shiseido is famous for its quality advertising.*

11

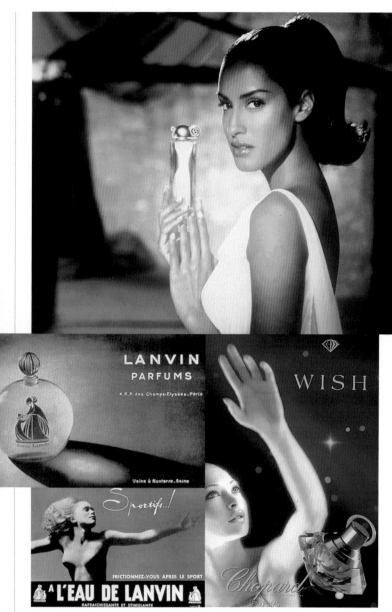

MIDDLE AND ABOVE: *1930s advertisements for Lanvin.*

TOP: *Organza, the most popular Givenchy fragrance.*
ABOVE: *Sparkling advertisement for Chopard's Wish.*

INGREDIENTS AND PROCESSES

Until late in the nineteenth century the preparation of liquid scents was almost entirely a matter of blending fragrant oils extracted from plants, although a few ingredients of animal origin were used as well. Sometimes this extraction was an easy operation, sometimes prolonged and the yield very small. Occasionally it was impossible, so the perfumer's skill would instead be directed toward mixing other fragrances together to provide a passing imitation of the original.

Most people will think of plant fragrances as the scent of flowers, but it is surprising how many different parts of a plant can produce fragrance. Essential oil, also called essence, is obtained from flowers, buds, leaves, stems, wood, fruit, seeds, bark, gum, and rhizomes. In some cases the whole of a plant contains fragrance; in other cases different essences can be conjured out of different parts of the same plant. The bitter (or Seville) orange tree, for example, provides both neroli and, by another process, orange-flower oil from its flowers, together with oil of bigarade from the fruit peel and oil of petitgrain from the leaves, twigs, and small, unripe fruits; all of these oils have a different fragrance and are used in perfumery.

Among flowers, those with the thickest petals contain the most oil and, with the exception of the rose, white flowers generally tend to be the most fragrant.

ABOVE: *Seventeen different rose fragrances are known to perfumers.*

Synthetic Fragrances

Over time more and more plants yielding essential oils have been discovered, so that the perfumer, primarily a chemist, must also be a botanist, with some 500 to 600 different usable plant fragrances at his or her disposal. But this quantity of perfume ingredients is nothing compared with the huge range of synthetic fragrances, with complicated chemical names, which the perfumer can now use. Here the number available is several thousand. They are not often mentioned by name when writing about perfumery—hexahydro hexamethyl cyclopentabenzopyran doesn't sound very romantic in a perfume context, but it has been widely used to synthesize the fragrance of musk. In Worth's Je Reviens it is indeed a chemical, amyl salicylate, that provides the key floral element in the fragrance.

Nowadays, chemical ingredients will usually form the majority of a perfume's constituent parts, providing not only fragrance but also the means of improving other fragrances, making them more compatible with each other or inducing them to last longer. Such chemicals are referred to as fixatives (see the Glossary on page 187). While we needn't say much about the chemicals (or synthetics) because the matter is a highly technical subject, one group has to be mentioned, and that is what are known as aldehydes. They're derived from alcohol and some natural plant materials, and were discovered at the end of the nineteenth century. They were first brought into perfumery by Ernest Beaux when he created Chanel No5. They have various uses: anisic aldehyde, for example, provides the scent of hawthorn; decylic aldehyde helps to reproduce the smell of violets; and they can give a fragrance a distinctive odor of its own and a new richness and strength. They must also be used extremely carefully and only in minute quantity—one drop of the raw material spilled accidentally on your clothing can make you smell unpleasant!

Animal Ingredients

The ability to make a perfume last is a key element in a perfumer's skill. These days older women often comment how the great classic perfumes seem to fade much more quickly than when they were young. One of the reasons for this is that modern perfumes are mostly made on a large commercial scale in a factory and no longer contain the rare animal ingredients which, besides being so powerful, were so long-lasting and such excellent fixatives.

The principal animal ingredients that were once staples of the top perfumers were:

Ambergris For centuries nobody knew its source; it is a substance excreted by a sperm whale after eating cuttle fish and found in lumps of varying size floating in tropical seas or washed ashore. It must be weathered for at least three years before use.

Musk Grains (or seeds) from a walnut-sized pod removed (harmlessly) from the male musk deer of the Himalayas. The strongest fragrance of all. A drop left on a handkerchief can last for 40 years.

Civet A butter-like secretion taken from a pouch under the tail of the civet cat, found in Ethiopia, Burma, and Thailand.

Castoreum (castor) A creamy, reddish-brown secretion taken from sacs on the beaver; used—at first by Arab perfumers—since the ninth century AD.

In their original state these ingredients are so powerful that they are quite nauseous—they must be enormously diluted before they become fragrant. But, in any event, on top of animal-rights objections, the available supply is far too inadequate for them to have any place in modern commercial perfume manufacture. Their use is confined to the specialist perfumer using older methods, and perfumes containing them will be extremely expensive. Nowadays, in the mainstream of commercial practice they are all synthesized.

We've already touched on the processes for extracting essential oils, but these need clearer definition. They are:

Distillation When plant material is placed in boiling water the essential oil containing the fragrance evaporates with the steam; the steam is then condensed back into water, where the oil floats on top and can be collected. The process may be repeated to obtain an even purer oil. Late in the nineteenth century the process was much improved with steam distillation, under which the steam was condensed in narrow pipes passing through cold water.

Extraction by volatile solvents Fragrant material is placed on a perforated metal plate in an "extractor" and a volatile solvent, such as ether, is passed over it and led into a still, where it condenses into a semisolid mass called "concrete." Concrete consists of essential oil plus a waxy substance known as stearoptene. The two can be separated by another technique using alcohol, leaving the oil in the purest and most concentrated form possible, termed as the "absolute." It is an extremely expensive product. Tuberose absolute, for example, now costs more than its weight in gold.

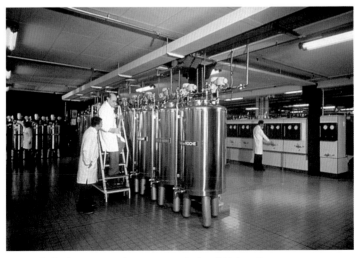

ABOVE: *Rochas' processing plant, computerized and high-tech.*

Enfleurage This is a technique used by the ancient Egyptians and continued right through to the twentieth century. By laying flower heads on oil or fat, which absorb fragrance, perfumers could take advantage of the fact that some flowers continue to produce essential oil for a while even after they have been picked. In France this was done commercially from the seventeenth century, particularly with jasmine, using sheets of glass coated with treated fat, which was then dissolved with alcohol to recover the oil. The method was extremely labor-intensive and is no longer used.

Expression This is the method usually used to obtain fragrant oil from the rinds of citrus fruits. The rinds are crushed between rollers and the oil is then separated by centrifugal force (in other words, spinning so that the oil is thrown out from the pulp).

There is one other way of making fragrant material for use in perfumery that has only recently been developed. It is a system called "head space technology," or "living-flower technology," and enables the fragrance of, in theory, virtually anything to be reproduced—a flower scent or, should you so want, the smell of old boots.

In effect, a fragrant object, say a flower head, is placed inside a special container and a vacuum is induced. For a while the flower will exude its scent inside the vacuum. After, say, half an hour the exudation is drawn off into a gas chromatograph machine, which exactly analyzes and measures the constituent elements of the fragrance exuded.

By assembling the same chemicals in the same proportions on a much larger scale, the fragrance can then be reproduced in much greater quantity. The technique is new, sometimes impossibly expensive, and presents many complications, but it has given perfumers an entirely new approach to perfume creation and many recent commercial perfumes now include fragrances made in this way.

BELOW: *"Head space technology" can be used to recreate the scent of any flower.*

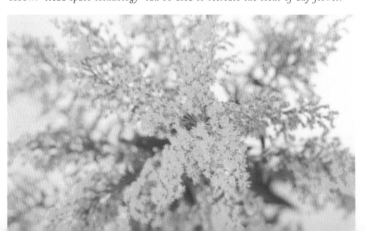

PRINCIPAL PERFUME PLANTS AND OILS

Balsam A resinous exudation from certain trees and shrubs, also called balm. In modern perfumery the principal ones used are balsam of Peru, of tolu, of Copaiba, and also storax. They all have a vanilla-like odor.

Bergamot An orange-scented oil expressed from the fruit peel of the bergamot orange tree. Used in about 33 percent of women's perfumes.

Bitter orange The oil of this name is obtained by expression from the fruit peel, the tree also being called Bigarade orange. The tree produces neroli, orange-flower oil, and petitgrain oil.

Frankincense (also Olibanum) A gum resin from small trees growing in South Arabia and Somalia. Very important since ancient times as an incense, for which it is still used. The Romans imported vast quantities of it. It is used as a main ingredient in about 13 percent of modern perfumes.

Galbanum A gum resin from a giant fennel found in Iran. It has a spicy-green, leaflike, musky odor.

Jasmine After rose this is the most important plant used in perfumery, appearing as a main ingredient in more than 80 percent of modern perfumes. Of several species, the Spanish or royal jasmine has been the most used in Europe since the sixteenth century. An acre of jasmine yields about 500 pounds of jasmine blossom, but the yield of absolute from that (at about 0.1 percent) is tiny, making jasmine one of the most expensive perfume materials available.

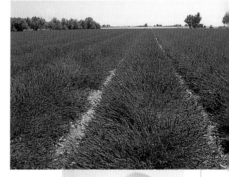

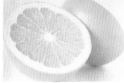

TOP: *Lavender*
ABOVE: *Lemon*

Labdanum (also called Ledanon). A sweet-scented oleo resin obtained in droplets from under the leaves of *Cistus* plants in the Middle East. Of great importance in perfumery, its fragrance resembles ambergris (it is often called amber) and it is a valuable fixative. Appears in about 33 percent of modern perfumes.

Lavender A major perfume material since Greek and Roman times. At one time France grew nearly 5,000 tons of flowers a year. In England production is now confined to Norfolk in the east. One acre produces about 15 pounds of oil.

Lemon Lemon oil, vital in flavorings as well as in perfumes, yields about a pound of oil to 1,000 lemons. The oil is expressed from the rinds and is used in

many quality perfumes, giving top notes a
fresh sparkle.

Lily of the Valley In early days this scent could
be obtained only by infusing the flowers in sweet
oils. Nowadays it is extracted as a concrete or
absolute and no essential oil is distilled. A synthetic is
then added and this produces the most exquisite lily
fragrance known, called muguet (this name is also used
as an alternative to lily of the valley). It is found in about
14 percent of all modern quality perfumes.

Myrrh A gum resin from myrrh trees, found in Arabia,
Somalia, and Ethiopia. Its use has been of great importance
since earliest times in medicine and embalming as well as in
perfumery, where it provides a balsamic note and is an excellent
fixative. It is found among the main ingredients of about 7 percent
of modern fine fragrances.

Neroli Steam-distilled from the flowers of the bitter orange tree
(brought to Europe by the Arabs in the twelfth century), this is
named after a sixteenth-century Italian prince whose wife scented
her bath and gloves with it. The odor combines spiciness with sweet and flowery
notes. A main ingredient in about 12
percent of all modern perfumes.

Oak moss A lichen taken from oak,
spruce, and other trees in mountain
areas of Europe and North Africa.
The fragrance develops when it is
stored and is earthy, woody, and
musky. Blending well and a good
fixative, it appears in a third of
present-day fine fragrances. See also
Tree moss.

Orris A butter-colored oil with a
violet-like fragrance extracted from
the rhizomes of certain species of
iris after they have been stored for

ABOVE: *Myrrh.*

two years. It has the unusual property of strengthening other fragrances.
Appears in many top perfumes.

Patchouli Most powerful of all plant materials. A Far-Eastern mintlike herb
with leaves which are dried and fermented before being distilled. The unique
odor of spice and cedar in this oil, which can be used only in minute quantities
because of its strength, actually improves with age. It is one of the finest
fixatives known. It first came to European notice in the nineteenth century,
when Indian traders exported shawls scented with it, which became highly
fashionable. Appears in a third of all top perfumes.

Rose The most important plant in perfumery since the earliest days of history. The Greek poet Sappho called it "the queen of the flowers." The cabbage rose, or painter's rose, known also as May rose, was the rose grown for perfume in France, but now many others are cultivated, while the Kazanlak district of Bulgaria produces huge quantities of the damask rose, and there is much cultivation in Egypt, Morocco, and elsewhere. Some 17 different rose scents have been identified. Nearly

ABOVE: *Rose—the most commonly used flower.*

1,000 pounds of roses are needed to distill just one pound of rose oil (attar or otto), and the yield of absolute from this is only around 0.03 percent. At least 75 percent of all quality perfumes contain rose oil.

Sandalwood This oil is distilled from the sawdust and chippings of the sandalwood tree of India and Indonesia, the very best coming from Mysore. The tree is parasitic, attaching suckers to other trees. One of the most valuable and expensive raw materials used in perfumery, very long-lasting and used in the base notes of about half of all quality perfumes.

Tonka Comes from angostura and para beans, produced by two species of a South American tree. These are cured in rum, when they become covered in crystals of coumarin, which smells of new-mown hay. The absolute extracted

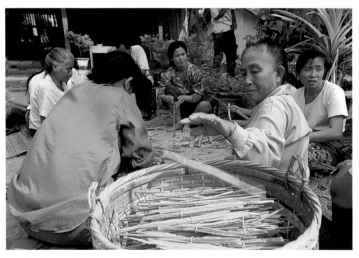

ABOVE: *Women chopping sticks of sandalwood.*

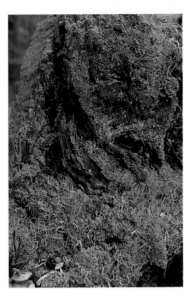

ABOVE: *Tree moss.*

from this is used in about 10 percent of all fine fragrances.

Tree moss In the USA tree moss and oak moss are the same. In European perfumery "tree moss" designates a lichen found on certain spruce and fir trees from which a resin with a powerfully tarlike odor is extracted. It is used especially in fougère and chypre perfumes and is a good fixative.

Tuberose With a fragrance described as that of a well-stocked flower garden in the evening, this oil, taken from the flower, appears in about 20 percent of quality perfumes. The yield of absolute is so small, however (about seven ounces for every 2,600 pounds or so of flowers) that it costs more than its weight in gold.

Vanilla Vanilla forms in crystals on the fruit pods of the vanilla orchid vine, native to Mexico and tropical America, which are picked and fermented. With a sweet spicy aroma, it became highly popular in perfumery after Coty introduced it in L'Aimant and now appears in a quarter of all fine perfumes.

Vetiver An oil distilled from the rhizomes of a tropical Asian grass called khus-khus. Has an earthy odor with underlying violet and orris-like sweetness. Long-lasting and a very good fixative. Appears in the base notes of 36 percent of quality perfumes.

Violet In perfumery two varieties of this plant are used, the Victoria, which has the better perfume, and the Parma, which is more easily grown. Oil is produced from the flowers and from the leaves of this plant, but it is so costly that most violet perfumes produced are now made synthetically.

Ylang-ylang This fragrance is used in some 40 percent of all quality perfumes. This oil is distilled from the leaves of the ylang-ylang tree

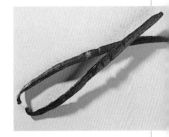

ABOVE: *Vanilla.*

of South East Asia. The powerful jasmine-like fragrance does not appear in the flowers until two weeks after they have opened, when they must be picked and distilled at once, so distillation is usually on site. One tree provides about 22 pounds of flowers a year and almost 900 pounds are needed for just two pounds of oil.

CLASSIFICATIONS AND CATEGORIES

The classification by scent of all the different fragrances has always been difficult; describing a smell is not easy. At the end of the nineteenth century Eugene Rimmel, a major London perfume-maker of French origin whose company still manufactures cosmetics, proposed splitting up the range of fragrances used in perfume into 18 groups (thus the sandal group would include sandalwood, vetiver, and cedarwood).

Around the same time another perfumer, Charles Piesse, tried to introduce the concept of arranging perfume odors on the basis of musical notes. He reckoned that an effective bouquet of fragrances could be achieved only with odors corresponding to a harmonious chord in music. The system failed, but the link with musical terms has remained, so we still talk of notes and chords.

William Poucher, in the 1920s, measured the evaporation rates of perfume materials against a scale of 100. It meant that the fragrances that evaporate most quickly and are most suitable as top notes—mandarin (one of the fastest evaporating of all), cilantro, lavender, bergamot, and mimosa, for example—appeared at the head of the scale; while the longest lasting—ambergris, balsam, labdanum, oak moss, frankincense, patchouli, sandalwood, tonka, and vetiver, for example—appeared among the base notes at the bottom.

The classification of individual fragrances has never gone much further than this and for ordinary purposes the tendency is simply to use a number of loose terms adopted over the years to describe individual notes. These include amber, aromatic, balsamic, camphoraceous, citrus, coniferous, crystalline, dry, earthy, floral, fougère, fruity, gourmand, green, hayfield (or haylike), herbaceous, heavy, leather, light, marine, metallic, minty, mossy, narcotic, oceanic, ozonic, powdery, smoky, sparkling, spicy, sweet, tobacco, and woody. More could be listed, and from time to time other such words come into use. For explanations of the less obvious ones see the Glossary on page 187.

The evaporation rate of fragrant oils is a key aspect of modern perfumery, because of the way perfumes are composed. Throughout history up to the end of the nineteenth century perfumers had produced single-note (single-fragrance) perfumes, which provided the scent of a specific plant or of a posy of plants.

The Pyramid System

Changes in the smell as evaporation caused different oils to fade at different rates were simply seen as part of the aging process. Then came the notion of building up the perfume on a more structured basis, brilliantly brought into effect by Aimé Guerlain with Jicky in 1889. Since then most commercial perfumes have been made on the pyramid (also three-tier, three-layer, or classical) system. These three tiers are its top, middle, and lower notes.

The top note (head note, head, or outgoing note) contains the most volatile of the perfume's ingredients. These will last for only a short time, perhaps no more than minutes, and are designed to attract attention and give a striking, quick, but concordant first impression. The middle note, also named the heart, rapidly supercedes the top note and reveals the main elements of the perfume. It is where the principal fragrances lie, supported by base notes, and should last at least four hours. The lower note (base note, back note, depth note, body note, dry-down, or dry-away) contains the longest-lasting (i.e. slowest-evaporating) fragrances, providing the perfume's fixatives and holding it all together. It may last for a day or more.

For convenience the description of a three-tier perfume, showing its principal plant ingredients, is very often written down in the shape of a pyramid, as in two examples here. The notes shown are the principal ones used in the making of the perfume, though by no means all. Aldehydes may be mentioned, but not normally any other chemical ingredient, since this is very much a guide for the layperson. When the absolute of an oil has been used, perfumers sometimes show this in the pyramid too ("tuberose abs.," for instance) as an indication that the perfume contains natural ingredients of exceptionally high (and expensive) quality.

PACO RABANNE'S **Calandre (1968)** (created by Michael Hy)	GUY LAROCHE'S **Fidji (1966)** (created by Josephine Catapano)
TOP NOTE — *bergamot* / *aldehydes*	*galbanum* / *ylang-ylang* — **HEAD**
MIDDLE NOTE — *rose, lily of the valley jasmine, gardenia ylang-ylang*	*Bulgarian rose jasmine tuberose, iris spices* — **HEART**
LOWER NOTE — *vetiver, oak moss sandalwood cedar, musk, amber, civet*	*ambergris, balsam musk, patchouli sandalwood* — **BASE**

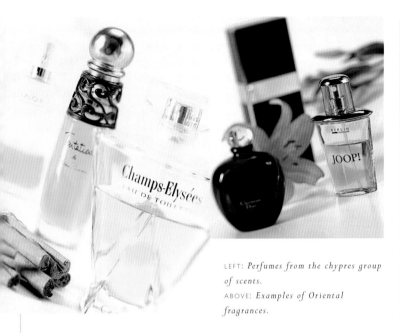

LEFT: *Perfumes from the chypres group of scents.*

ABOVE: *Examples of Oriental fragrances.*

Fragrance Groups

With thousands of perfumes on the market, there is an obvious need to sort them into categories in some way. This is usually done by separating them into what are known as family groups, also called fragrance groups or just categories (as in this book). Four family groups have commonly been recognized for a long time—**floral**, **chypre**, **amber** (oriental), and **fougère**—and, with increasing varieties of fragrance coming into use, these have been both sub-divided and added to.

In recent years the august French Society of Perfumers has tried to standardize the system and has defined the main families as **citrus** (Hesperidic), **floral**, **fougère**, **chypre**, **woody**, **amber** (oriental), and **leather**, all of them much subdivided.

However, no universally acknowledged categorization has emerged. With perfumes containing many fragrances they may even be discerned differently by different people, when there can be some apparent contradiction of category under different systems. The French system is shown on pages 24–25, but in the main part of this book the categories are mostly those notified by the companies concerned and may differ.

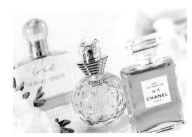

RIGHT: *Floral fragrances.*

the perfume families

(Note: *m = fragrances in this subdivision are mostly or entirely masculine*)

FAMILY	SUBDIVISIONS	EXAMPLES
A. Citrus (Hesperidic)	**1.** Citrus (m)	*Eau de Patou*
	2. Floral chypre citrus	*Ô de Lancôme, Eau de Rochas*
	3. Citrus spicy (m)	
	4. Citrus woody (m)	
	5. Citrus aromatic (m)	*Eau de Courrèges*
B. Floral	**1.** Single flower	*(All single-flower fragrances)*
	2. Lavender single flower (m)	
	3. Floral bouquet	*Quelques Fleurs, Je Reviens, Joy, Anaïs-Anaïs, Giorgio, Eternity, Trésor*
	4. Floral green	*Vent Vert, Chanel No. 19, Safari*
	5. Floral aldehydic	*Chanel No 5, L'Aimant, Loulou*
	6. Floral woody (m)	
	7. Floral fruity woody	*Nahema, Armani, Tiffany, Kenzo*
C. Fougère	**1.** Fougère	*Jicky, Canoe*
	2. Soft amber fougère (m)	
	3. Floral amber fougère (m)	
	4. Spicy fougère (m)	
	5. Aromatic fougère (m)	

FAMILY	SUBDIVISIONS	EXAMPLES
D. Chypre	**1.** Chypre	*Chypre*
	2. Floral chypre (m)	
	3. Floral aldehydic chypre	*Ma Griffe, Paloma Picasso, Knowing*
	4. Fruity chypre	*Mitsouko, Y, V'E, Cristalle, Femme*
	5. Green chypre	*Miss Dior, Givenchy III*
	6. Aromatic chypre (m)	
	7. Leather chypre	*Jolie Madame, Miss Balmain,*
		Montana, Cabochard, La Nuit
E. Woody	**1.** Woody (m)	
	2. Woody hesperidic coniferous (m)	
	3. Woody aromatic (m)	
	4. Woody spicy (m)	
	5. Woody spicy leather (m)	
	6. Woody amber (m)	
F. Amber (oriental)	**1.** Floral woody amber	*Shocking, Bijan, Passion, Joop!, Habanita, Samsara*
	2. Floral spicy amber	*L'Heure Bleue, Soir de Paris, Poison, Vol de Nuit, Byzance, Red Door*
	3. Soft amber	*Tabu, Chantilly, Shalimar*
	4. Citrus amber (m)	
	5. Floral semi-amber	*Youth Dew, Opium, Coco, Gem, Boucheron*
G. Leather	**1.** Leather	*Tabac Blond, Cuir de Russie, Scandale*
	2. Floral leather (m)	
	3. Tobacco leather (m)	

CREATION AND MANUFACTURE

These days most professional perfumers (the "noses") learn their art at institutions such as the famous Givaudan-Roure School of Perfumery in Grasse, where a full course, including field training and a period of apprenticeship with a manufacturer, takes six years. It used to be the case that almost all "noses" were men (Germaine Cellier, creator of the classic Vent Vert for Balmain, being one of the few exceptions). Now there are many women in the top ranks of perfumery, and the proportion of men to women has almost evened out.

Creation may be the highest art of perfumers, but they also have more practical duties. For example, a perfume that is to be sold over many years must be reblended as supplies are used up, and the perfumer must ensure that the aroma of the new materials exactly matches the originals, whatever the effect of droughts and diseases on crops.

Health and Safety

The industry as a whole is very alert to the risks of using powerful oils: ingredients must conform with international regulations laid down for environmental or health reasons and many materials, including synthetics, can no longer be used without chemical modification, or have had to be replaced altogether, because some trace of toxicity has been found in them. Many

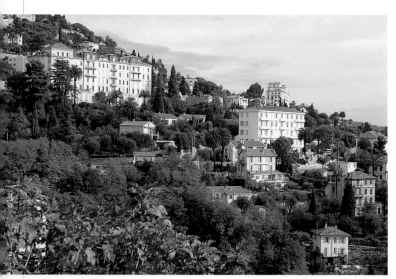

ABOVE: *Grasse—center of the European perfume industry.*

perfumers will be engaged on this sort of work or on devising simple fragrances for soaps, cleaning fluids, and room fresheners rather than creating new Diorissimos and L'Air du Temps for the fine-fragrance market.

The decision to create and launch a new perfume on the world market is a hard commercial undertaking, usually based on market research and requiring very substantial financial support. Problems of type and cost must be settled at an early stage, quite possibly before the "nose" comes into the reckoning at all. A sale price must be determined, a ceiling placed on the cost of advertising and marketing, the image the company seeks to convey with its product must be agreed. Most important, an appropriate bottle must be found. Surprisingly often, the whole project begins with nothing but the perfume's name.

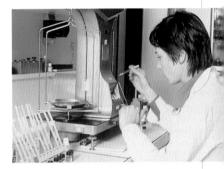

Nowadays almost all perfumers, except those who have set up their own small businesses making and selling their own perfumes (like Nicolaï and Isabell),

ABOVE: *A perfumer testing fragrant oils.*

work for one or two of the very big fragrance manufacturing companies. Only a few of the very largest perfume houses—for example Guerlain, Chanel, Patou—have their own "noses" any more and, with one or two exceptions like Guy Robert (creator of perfumes such as Madame Rochas and Gucci No. 1), no prominent, independent "noses" are left.

As the criteria for the proposed new perfume become more definite, a manufacturing company, or very probably more than one, will be approached. Samples are provided, changes considered, until at last, a selection is made, and a "nose" is chosen to take on the creation.

Sitting (sometimes) at his "organ," a desk surrounded by shelves full of bottles containing basic essential oils and synthetic preparations, the perfumer attempts by degrees to build up the required fragrance. He or she will have needed years of experience to learn the hundreds of different aromas that can be brought into his blend, the effect one fragrance may have on another, how to sharpen a fragrance or ensure one element does not overwhelm another. The final product may contain something of the perfumer's own style—a preference for one ingredient, even a favorite accord introduced as a personal signature— but above all it must meet the wishes of the client, which can sometimes be very difficult to interpret.

Ernest Daltroff cannot have been too pleased when an eccentric American millionaire asked him to create a scent that would raise the memory of having a bath in champagne—but Caron still sells Royal Bain de Champagne, which has subsequently found another use in voodoo rituals!

Nor for that matter can Jacques Cavallier of Firmenich have felt too confident about creating Issey Miyake's first fragrance when the only requirement obtainable from the designer was that it should smell like fresh water! But L'Eau d'Issey has become a bestseller.

No perfume can be tested quickly. A few sniffs and the nose tires, so there may be hours, or even days, between one test and the next. Scientific testing may be needed to ensure that the aroma will last long enough on the skin. The client may even want a judgment from his own panel, perhaps leading to further modifications. The process of getting a perfume onto the market can therefore take years and has certainly never been a hurried matter. But not many will drag their heels these days as long as Coty's L'Aimant, which took five years to perfect, or Guerlain's Chant d'Arômes, which was under preparation for seven!

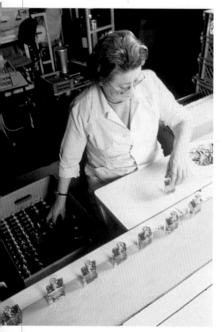

ABOVE: *Quality control—every bottle must be perfect.*

The Quantity of Quality

Professional perfumers are constructing extremely elaborate concoctions. Most perfumes contain 50 to 100 ingredients, but others have many more: 200 is quite normal. Wings, by Giorgio Beverly Hills, is claimed to have 621, and Red, from the same house, nearly 700. The great majority of these ingredients are chemicals, many of which will have been extracted from plants, but others may originate from tar, petroleum, and other seemingly unlikely sources.

The very quantity of ingredients to be handled requires an elaborate and, in these high-tech days, highly computerized organization to hold, store correctly, and control them; their preparation into a full-scale commercial perfume needs the resources of a major manufacturer.

Manufacture within the perfume industry starts with the preparation of all the many different essential oils. Some of this may be done centrally, but much of it is undertaken in distant locations. Thus, the flowers of the ylang-ylang tree from southeast Asia must be picked at a precise moment in their development and distilled immediately, so the distillery has to be close to the trees, the oil then being shipped onward in vats. This means that a perfume manufacturer must either run its own distillery on the site or purchase the oil wholesale from a local owner or another manufacturer.

Then there is the process of assembling and blending together all the ingredients of the perfume in conformity with the formula produced by the "nose." These ingredients are mixed into a concentrate which is left for several weeks to blend, then diluted in alcohol to the required strength and kept in copper containers to mature. Only then is it bottled ready for the launch.

Fragrance is now a very large-scale business, used not only in perfumes but in all sorts of household preparations from soaps to lavatory cleaners. It is also closely allied to flavor, for it is the smell of a tasty dish that makes you want to eat it, and flavorings often come from the same ingredients. There are now huge companies, with branches all over the world, manufacturing both fragrances and flavors. These and a few smaller fragrance-manufacturing companies employ most of the perfumers.

But many perfumers still operate outside of this great international industry, making fragrances in small laboratories and selling them from their own small stores. From here can be obtained the rarities: perfumes made with aloewood or ambergris; perfumes designed for a minority taste; perfumes with unusual effects, or exclusive individual perfumes for connoisseurs, like The Scent of Romance, created by John Bailey of the Perfumers Guild for the British writer Barbara Cartland.

Most of these rely almost wholly on natural ingredients and, through both the fragrances and the atmosphere of the stores, will take one nearer to those days when the first of the Guerlains, creating delicate scents to suit the mood of perhaps just a single evening, began to turn perfumery into a new art form.

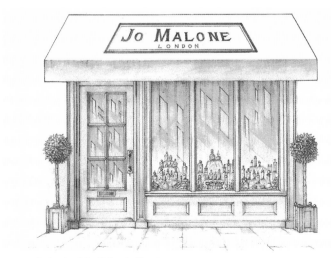

ABOVE: *A sketch of Jo Malone's flagship store.*

leading perfumers of today

NAME	PRESENT COMPANY	EXAMPLE CREATIONS
Almairac, Michel	Drom	*Heaven, Casmir*
Anthony, Gérard	Drom	*Nilang, XS pour Elle*
Apel, David	Fragrance Resources	*Sunflowers, Luciano Pavarotti*
Bourdon, Pierre	Fragrance Resources	*Dolce Vita, Cool Water*
Buxton, Marc	Créations Aromatiques	*Dalissime, Comme des* Garçons
Caron, Françoise	Quest	*Just Me, Gio, Kenzo, Madeleine Vionnet*
Cavallier, Jacques	Firmenich	*L'Eau D'Issey, Poême, Alchimie*
Cresp, Olivier	Firmenich	*Angel, L'Eau per Kenzo*
Delville, Jean-Claude	IFF	*Cabotine, Wings*
Ellena, Bernard	Dragoco	*Tribu, Hanae Mori*
Ellena, Jean-Claude	Haarmann & Reimer	*First, Bvlgari, Un Matin d'Été*
Feisthauer, Nathalie	Givaudan-Roure	*Eau Belle, Nuits Indiennes, Blonde*
Fléchier, Edouard	Givaudan-Roure	*Tendre Poison, Parfum de Peau*
Grosjman, Sophia	IFF	*Eternity, Yvresse, Jaipur, Trésor, Spellbound, Sun Moon Stars, Paris, Lalique, White Diamonds*
Guerlain, Jean-Paul	Guerlain	*Guerlain fragrances*
Guichard, Jean	Givaudan-Roure	*Poison, Obsession, Loulou, Eden, Deci Dela, So Pretty*
Kerleo, Jean	Patou	*Patou fragrances, Yohji*
Labbé, Sophie	IFF	*Organza, Jardins de Soleil, Folie Douce, Iceberg for Her*
Latty, Jean-François	Takasago	*Love Story*
Lorson, Nathalie	IFF	*Romeo Gigli, Folie Douce, Wish*
Ménardeau, Annick	Firmenich	*Eau d'Eden, Lolita Lempicka*
Nagel, Christine	Quest	*Une Nuite Étoilée au Bengal*
Pellegrino, Roger	Firmenich	*Anaïs-Anaïs, Gem, Léonard*
Polge, Jacques	Chanel	*Chanel perfumes*
Preyssas, Dominique	Takasago	*Basala, Talisman*
Robert, François	Dragoco	*Apogée, La Rose de Rosine*

NAME	PRESENT COMPANY	EXAMPLE CREATIONS
Robert, Guy	independent	*Amouage, Calèche, Gucci No 1, Dioressence*
Roche, Daniella	Givaudan-Roure	*Io La Perla, Very Velentino*
Ropion, Dominique	Haarmann & Reimer	*Ysatis, Amarige, Aimez-Moi, Jungle*
Roucel, Maurice	Dragoco	*Tocade, 24 Faubourg, Monsoon*
Sheldrake, Christopher	Quest	*Féminité du Bois, Toccadilly*
Sieuzac, Jean-Louis	Haarmann & Reimer	*Opium, Dune, Aimez-Moi*

(Note: *As in any industry, perfumers change jobs from one company to another, so some of the above examples of their creations may have been for a different company.*)

leading perfume manufacturers

COMPANY	EMPLOYEES (worldwide, approx.)	HEADQUARTERS
Bush Boake Allen	2,500	*Montvale, NJ, USA*
Créations Aromatiques	180	*Geneva, Switzerland*
Charabot	374	*Grasse, France*
Dragoco	1,800	*Holzminden, Germany*
Drom Fragrances International	180	*Munich, Germany*
Firmenich	3,000	*Geneva, Switzerland*
Fragrances Resources	160	*La Tour de Peilz, Switzerland*
Givaudan-Roure	5,300	*Verrier, Switzerland*
Haarmann & Reimer-Florasynth	5,400	*Holzminden, Germany*
International Flavors & Fragrances (IFF)	4,600	*New York, USA*
Mane	1,100	*La Bar sur Loup, France*
Quest	4,500	*Colombes, France*
Robertet	800	*Grasse, France*
Takasago	2,200	*Tokyo, Japan*

BOTTLES AND DESIGNERS

Sometime during the fourth millennium BC (you could almost say "once upon a time") the ancient Egyptians discovered how to manufacture glass, and over the centuries they developed a technique for making containers by coating a clay core on the end of a metal rod with molten glass and scraping out the core once the glass had cooled and hardened.

By about 1500 BC quite skillfully made glass perfume bottles were in use, mostly in dark-blue, opaque, or translucent glass decorated with zigzag stripes of blue, white, or yellow—the Lalique flacons of the age.

We may be sure that at that time a glass scent bottle was a great luxury, as were its contents, but perfumes had been made and kept in containers for hundreds of years already. These earlier containers were originally produced in terra cotta, highly porous for a precious liquid, and later, for the wealthy, carved out of alabaster, onyx, and porphyry, which had the great merit of being able to keep unguents cool and so delay the time when their fatty contents would begin to go rancid.

Greeks and Romans

All these substances continued in use in Greek and Roman times, but in designs that became increasingly more sophisticated. Many Greek scent bottles have been found of pottery made in the shape of birds, and animal or human heads.

In about 50 BC the development in Syria of glass-blowing—enabling glass to be shaped before it had cooled—was a huge technological stride, the more so when the method was refined by blowing the glass into a mold, so that production of the same item could be repeated. Roman scent bottles of transparent glass with colored glass decoration

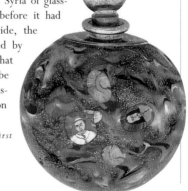

ABOVE: *Glass bottle for balsam (Scythian, first century BC).*
RIGHT: *Gilded, molded glass bottle used for Molinard's Habanita fragrance, c. 1923.*

and in a wide variety of shapes and designs often display a remarkably high standard of craftsmanship. But these were expensive; most citizens kept their simple unguents in containers, very often shell-shaped, made of earthenware.

In the Middle Ages metal and enamelware appeared, but beyond these it was not until the eighteenth century that any significant new material became available for making scent bottles, when the Chinese secret of manufacturing porcelain was discovered. From factories in Meissen in Germany, Sèvres in France, Chelsea in England, and eventually scores of other centers, little decorative porcelain scent bottles began to appear on the dressing tables of fashionable homes.

But glass remained the preeminent material for perfume containers. For one thing, the powerful oils in the fragrance could react to porcelain, and vice versa; for another, it was difficult to make a stopper in porcelain that provided a totally reliable seal, essential for any manufacturer on a large scale.

The Age of the Bottle

Until about the end of the nineteenth century perfume was sold by the perfumer in plain containers and decanted into scent bottles in the home, or a customer might choose a scent and select a bottle at the same time. This led to stores selling a vast range of beautiful perfume bottles designed to please every personal taste.

But, when perfume-makers began to produce their wares in the sophisticated pyramid style of modern perfumery it had to be bottled in a factory. A key feature of the bottle was that it should attract a would-be purchaser.

We owe it to a few influential people in the perfume industry at that time, in particular François Coty, that the bottles that set the standards from the very start of factory-produced perfume were designed to a very high quality with exquisite taste by master craftsmen—Lalique, and Baccarat, but Maurice Martinot, Lucien Gaillard, Süe et Mare, Maurice Dépinoix, and Viard et Viollet le Duc are but a few of those who produced wonderful designs over the next decades. With a growing number of scent-bottle collectors, their work now commands huge prices at auction.

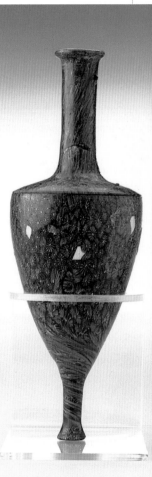

ABOVE: *Blown amethyst glass bottle, 50–150 AD.*

The appearance of the bottle is a vital factor in selling a perfume, and these days all the big perfume houses employ top-class bottle designers, sometimes their own, more often one of the surprisingly few freelance designers who work in this part of the art world. The doyen of these is Pierre Dinand. Their designs are put into effect in hundreds of thousands by the big specialist glassmakers, who may also have their own designers, such as Brosse, Saint Gobain Desjonquères, BSN Verreries de Manières, Pochet et du Courval, and Luigi Bormioli in Europe, and Wheaton Glassworks and Carr-Lowry in the USA.

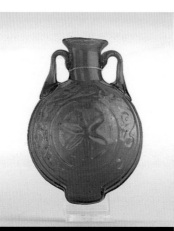

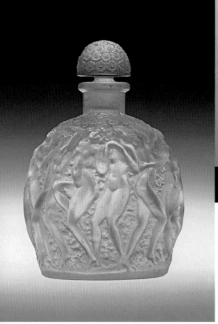

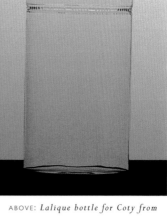

ABOVE: *Lalique bottle for Coty from the 1920s.*

LEFT: *Molded, frosted glass bottle designed by René Lalique for Molinard.*

TOP LEFT: *Mold blown glass jar, dating from the Roman Empire, first century AD.*

contemporary perfume-bottle designers

DESIGNER	EXAMPLES
Fabien Baron	CK One, Poême, 212 Carolina Herrera, Innocence, Contradiction, Jil, CK Be
Thierry de Baschmakoff	Bvlgari pour Femme, Popy Moreni, Yohji, Just Me, Madeleine Vionnet, Face à Face
Annagret Beier	bottles for Cacharel
Pierre Davene	bottles for Givenchy
Joël Desgrippes	Amazone, Boucheron, Calèche, So Pretty, Jungle, Magic
Pierre Dinand	Bal à Versailles, Escape, Iceberg Twice, Obsession, Opium, Nicole Miller, Ysatis, Rive Gauche, Volupté, Madame Rochas, Yvresse
Robert Granai	bottles for Guerlain
Jacques Helleu	bottles for Chanel
Bernard Kotyuk	Escada, Vanderbilt, Sunny Frutti
Thierry Lecoule	Cabotine, V'E, Stradivarius d'Arman
Ira Levy	bottles for Estée Lauder
Serge Mansau	Blonde, Diorella, Dolce Vita, Infini, Kenzo, 24 Faubourg, Organza, Parfum d'Été, Tocade, Folie Douce, Alchimie, Toccadilly, Love Story
Alain de Morgues	Accenti, Paris, Quelques Fleurs, Raffinée, L'Eau d'Issey, Lolita Lempicka, Sonia Rykiel
Frederico Restrepo	Baroque, Etiquette Bleu, Baccarat, Aimez-Moi
Peter Schmidt	Gucci No 3, Joop Femme, Venezia, Hugo Woman, All About Eve, Cool Water Woman
Susan Wacker	bottles for Elizabeth Arden

CHOOSING
AND USING

Perfume, in its strictest sense, is a blend of fragrant oils diluted in a high-grade alcohol in a concentration containing about 15–20 percent oil, the alcohol being about 90–95 percent pure. This is a *parfum*, also known as an *extrait* or extract. Any mixture with a lower proportion of oil to alcohol is an *eau* (water).

There are different strengths of *eau*, principally *eau de parfum,* with 15-18 percent of oil mixed in a slightly weaker alcohol, *eau de toilette* (4-8 percent of oil in an even weaker alcohol); and *eau de cologne* (3-5 percent of oil in a still weaker oil/alcohol mix). Recently *eau fraîche* has come into use, which is a cologne with a purer alcohol. Sometimes the mixtures go outside of these percentages.

Most perfumes come in a line which contains a *parfum* or *eau de parfum* (or both) as well as an *eau de toilette*, but sometimes the highest available concentration is only at *eau de toilette* strength. The line may also contain body lotions, soaps, bath foams, and so on, but these are just toilet preparations to which a small dash of the fragrance has been added.

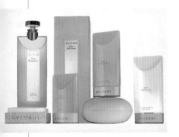

ABOVE: *Bvlgari's Eau Parfumée product range.*

The question sometimes arises of where best to purchase a perfume. It is difficult to give advice on this, as everybody's circumstances are so different. You will not find a fully comprehensive range of perfumes anywhere, as there are so many on the market that retailers themselves have to be selective. If you have decided exactly what you want, then you might as well get it from the cheapest source you can find, always bearing in mind that if you buy on the sidewalk it will probably be a fake which ceases to exude fragrance after about ten minutes!

The connoisseur who likes to make a careful choice would do well to go somewhere that offers both a good range of products and good advice. In subtle ways different perfumes suit different people, so selecting what to buy is a matter of personal preference and taste, but there are trained consultants behind the counters of the larger department stores and the specialist perfumeries who can be very helpful and may save you a lot of time.

For a real experience, however, try the store of a perfumer selling his or her own creations. Buy a small bottle, to reduce the chance of its going stale before you've finished it.

Always try a fragrance on your own skin, but preferably not if you have just been eating strongly flavored food, or vigorously exercising, or if you have not quite recovered from an illness, feel out of sorts, or have just been smoking. All of these can affect the fragrance or your appreciation of it. Test an *eau de toilette* version of the perfume rather than any stronger concentration. Take a very small sample and don't rub it into the skin. The best point to apply it is on the wrist; you can then put a different perfume on the other wrist and, if needed, two more on either upper arm. Try to wait at least 20 minutes, preferably an hour, before deciding, so that the notes unfold.

Some perfumeries now provide blotting-paper wands on which to apply the fragrance; these may be useful as a first stage, since you can test several different fragrances with them, but they are no substitute for your skin in the final selection.

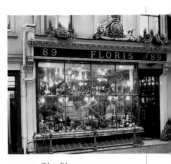

ABOVE: *The Floris company have been in London's Jermyn Street since 1730.*

Perfume lasts longest when applied to the pulse points, so your wrists, navel, collarbone area, or even behind the knees, are good places when you come to wear it—not behind the ears though, as the alcohol dries too quickly there. Some people find it lasts longer if sprayed on after a shower or bath, when the skin is still slightly damp.

There are also people who like to layer fragrances, especially for evening wear—use the soap and bath foam of the fragrance line at first, then the body lotion, finally apply the perfume itself; this may be expensively luxurious, but you will end up gorgeously fragrant.

Perfume is affected by air, heat, and light, so try to keep your bottle closed in a cool, dark place. Unopened, it may last 20 years, but once you have let air get in it will start to deteriorate and become acidic, the top notes going first. The more air, the worse the effect, so once opened it is really best to use it all within a year or two—and that, of course, will give you every excuse to choose a replacement without delay!

BELOW: *Bottle designs may vary with the different fragrance concentrations.*

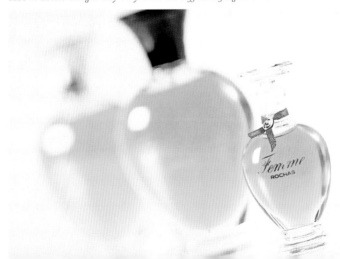

There are literally hundreds of perfume houses producing thousands of perfumes around the world. For reasons of space, this directory concentrates on perfumes for women, covering a range of small perfume houses to world-famous producers. The economics of the industry are changing. More fragrances are coming out on the international market than ever before—some two or three hundred a year. Some will be successful, but many will fail and disappear. The constantly changing whims of fashion play a major part in this. Competition and a variety of commercial pressures can create acute problems of survival and nowadays firms are constantly being taken over by others. Sometimes there may in fact be virtually nothing left of a distinguished perfume house except its reputation and the right, bought by a license, to use its name and to create and sell its perfumes. Arbitrary choices had to be made about which houses to include or omit. A company's exclusion is not a criticism of it or its products.

The entries are in alphabetical order (if the company title is a person's name it has been alphabetized by surname). Each entry gives an overview of the history of the company and of the people associated with it. The information contained within the fact box is as up to date as possible, detailing the name of the parent company, the location of their headquarters, and the current range of perfumes that are available (n/a indicates that the information was not available). There are feature perfumes detailed for each house, with information on when it was launched, the creator of the fragrance and the flacon, and the notes of the perfume. Unless otherwise stated the name of the designer of the original flacon has been given, although in some cases it has not been possible to show the original flacon.

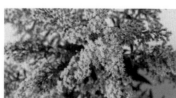
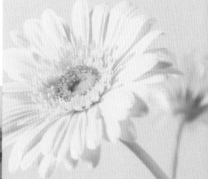

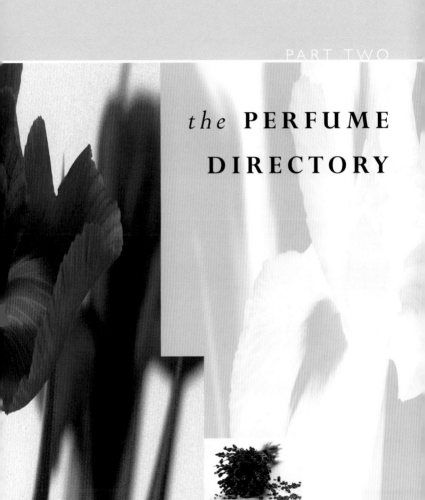

the **PERFUME
DIRECTORY**

AMOUAGE

Redolent of the Orient ... "the most valuable perfume in the world"

PARENT COMPANY	*independent*
HEADQUARTERS	*Seeb, Muskat, Sultanate of Oman*
CURRENT PERFUMES	*Amouage, Ubar*

If you want one of the real perfumes of Arabia, this is it. It was launched by a young Omani businessman, Sayyid Badr al Hamood, who wanted to revive Arabia's ancient association with luxurious fragrances. He enlisted the help of one of France's leading perfumers, Guy Robert, the "nose" for classics such as Madame Rochas, Dioressence, and Gucci No. 1, and asked for a perfume of Western style but redolent of the Orient, including sensuous Arabian ingredients like frankincense and myrrh.

The spectacular result was Amouage (pronounced "amwaaj"), which in Arabic signifies "waves of emotion." Called "the most valuable perfume in the world," it has over 120 natural ingredients and is contained in a range of expensive flacons of Islamic design, some in gilded silver and crystal. Since 1984 it has been selling widely in duty-free and the more prestigious stores. In 1995 the company followed up its success with a high-quality chypre perfume called Ubar, the name of a legendary Arabian city.

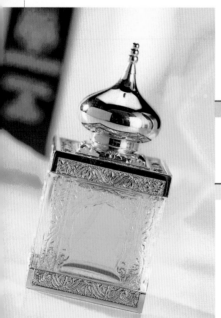

Amouage

LAUNCHED	*1984*
CREATOR	*Guy Robert*
CATEGORY	*floral oriental*
FLACON	*Brosse and others*

notes

TOP	*jasmine, rose, tuberose, orris, peach*
MIDDLE	*patchouli, labdanum, myrrh, frankincense, sandalwood, ylang-ylang*
LOWER	*musk, civet, ambergris*

ANTONIA'S FLOWERS

The distinctive fragrance of a flower store in summer

PARENT COMPANY	*independent*
HEADQUARTERS	*Massachusetts, USA*
CURRENT PERFUME	*Antonia's Flowers*

Antonia Bellanca was an art student who set up a little floral-design business in New York's exclusive East Hampton in 1981. She was soon the leading florist in the district, with famous residents like Estée Lauder and Calvin Klein among her clients.

Surrounded with flowers, Antonia found she could distinguish their individual scents but was unable to find any perfume that evoked the distinctive fragrance of a flower store in summer. This became a challenge and, with help from a leading perfumer, she set out to create one. It was just for herself but attracted so much attention that she decided to sell it in the store and found she had an instant hit.

Soon Antonia's Flowers, the perfume, replaced the flower store. By 1985 her perfume was among the ten best-selling fragrances in New York's famous Bergdorf Goodman store. Now it is sold throughout the US and internationally as well.

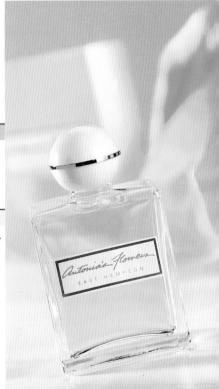

Antonia's Flowers

LAUNCHED	*1982*
CREATOR	*Antonia Bellanca*
CATEGORY	*floral*
FLACON	*confidential*

notes

TOP	*heady bouquet of freesia, jasmine, and magnolia, interspersed with fresh cuts of lily*
MIDDLE	*sweet, fruity*
LOWER	*sandalwood and subtle musky notes*

ELIZABETH ARDEN

A house of many fragrances—"beauty should be a combination of nature and science"

PARENT COMPANY	*Unilever*
HEADQUARTERS	*New York, USA*
CURRENT PERFUMES	*Blue Grass, Red Door, Sunflowers, 5th Avenue, Splendor*

The founder of Elizabeth Arden was Florence Nightingale Graham, a Canadian-American of British parentage born in Toronto, who started work with a cosmetics company in New York. She opened her own beauty salon on Fifth Avenue in 1910 and never looked back. The name, some say, was derived from a well-known book of that time, *Elizabeth and her German Garden*, but others believe she took the name from a combination of Tennyson's poem *Enoch Arden* and her own love of the name Elizabeth.

Whatever the answer, the signature bright-red front doors and distinctive pink interior decoration of her stores quickly became known widely. In a very short time she had introduced more cosmetic preparations than any other manufacturer. By 1932, when she launched her first range of varicolored lipsticks, she already had 29 stores around the world.

Miss Arden, as she became known, was indefatigable, with a demanding passion for detail, and, when she died in 1966 at the age of 83, she had

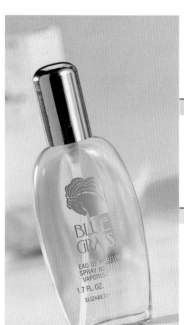

Blue Grass

LAUNCHED	*1936 (relaunched 1989)*
CREATOR	*George Fuchs (Fragonard)*
CATEGORY	*floral*
FLACON	*Denise Paglina (redesign)*

notes

TOP	*lavender, bergamot, orange flower*
MIDDLE	*jasmine, rose, lavender, spices*
LOWER	*sandalwood, vetiver, cedar*

Red Door

LAUNCHED *1989*
CREATOR *Claire Cain*
CATEGORY *floral*
FLACON *Denise Paglina*

notes

TOP *rose, violet, ylang-ylang*
MIDDLE *orchid, jasmine, lily of the valley, freesia, orange flower*
LOWER *vetiver, honey, woody notes*

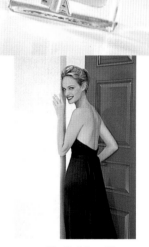

already been rewarded with royal warrants from the British Queen and Queen Mother.

At the beginning she sold perfumes by other makers. Her first house perfumes date from around 1922 with single-flower fragrances such as Arden Rose and Italian Lilac. In 1936 she brought out the immensely successful Blue Grass, now a classic, which was named to recall the view from the home in Virginia where she kept her horses. It was created for her by George Fuchs, the owner of Fragonard, who still makes perfumes in Grasse.

Of many other perfumes in the 1930s and 1940s should be noted two with magnificent Baccarat flacons now eagerly collected— Cyclamen, in a fan-shaped bottle which also offered a detachable jeweled pin, and It's You, in which the flacon is itself offered by a crystal hand. Altogether the company has issued well over 50 perfumes.

ABOVE: *The Red Door Woman is intriguing.*

When Elizabeth Arden died, the family connections with her company went too, and in 1971 it was purchased by the pharmaceutical giant Eli Lilly & Co., which brought new technical resources into the business. Miss Arden had always maintained that "beauty should be a combination of nature and science." There have been many subsequent corporate changes. In the 1970s the company was closely tied with the House of Chloé in Paris, France, and its prominent designer Karl Lagerfeld, leading to the launch of the perfumes Chloé and KL. From a link with Italy's Fendi sisters emerged the fragrance Fendi.

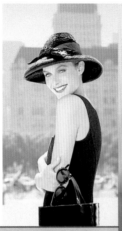

5th Avenue

LAUNCHED *1996*
CREATOR *Ann Gottlieb (IFF)*
CATEGORY *floral semi-oriental*
FLACON *Susan Wacker*

notes

TOP *lilac, linden, magnolia, muguet, mandarin, bergamot*

MIDDLE *rose, violet, ylang-ylang, tuberose, peach, clove, nutmeg*

LOWER *amber, musk, sandalwood, iris, vanilla*

ABOVE: *5th Avenue, for a woman with a style all her own.*

The company's collection of other fragrances includes White Diamonds by Elizabeth Taylor, Nino Cerruti, and Valentino. In 1987 Elizabeth Arden was itself bought by Fabergé, from whom Unilever acquired it two years later. There are now two fragrance companies under the control of Unilever: Elizabeth Arden, continuing its normal business, and a subsidiary called Parfums International, through which Elizabeth Arden runs the other perfume houses.

Apart from Blue Grass, Elizabeth Arden's own range of fragrances at present contains Red Door, a full *parfum* of rich floral notes contained in a bright red-domed bottle with a charm tied to it and relaunched using the model Linda Evangelista. The award-winning Sunflowers, advertised as "a celebration of life," is designed for younger women to wear during summery days. 5th Avenue, also a full *parfum*, has a classically elegant style in a modern setting, with its bottle design inspired by the New York skyline. A new fragrance, Splendor has been launched replacing True Love.

ARMANI

The fashion house with a nose for award-winning fragrances

PARENT COMPANY	*L'Oréal*
HEADQUARTERS	*Milan, Italy*
CURRENT PERFUMES	*Gio, Acqua di Gio, Emporio Armani for Her*

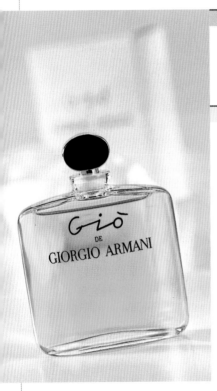

Gio

LAUNCHED	*1992*
CREATOR	*Françoise Caron (Givaudan-Roure)*
CATEGORY	*floral fruity*
FLACON	*Michel Blanc*

notes

TOP	*rose, hyacinth, jasmine*
MIDDLE	*iris, gardenia, orange blossom, tuberose, peach*
LOWER	*sandalwood, vanilla*

Compile a list of the world's most prominent designers of couture clothing and accessories for both men and women and you would undoubtedly have to include Giorgio Armani. He was born in 1934 in Piacenze, Northern Italy, but his base is the great Italian fashion center of Milan, where he set up his business and presented his first collection in 1974.

In 1982 Armani launched his first women's fragrance, Armani, a green floral in a smart octagonal bottle. Ten years later he followed this with Gio, a fresh fruity floral, which won a FiFi award (the "Oscars" of the fragrance industry) for best fragrance for women in 1994; it appeared in a bottle inspired by the classic wide-shouldered Armani suit. The simplicity of the bottle and the type reflects the Armani motto of "less is more." Acqua di Gio, an "aqua floral" designed to evoke the feeling of a summer's day in the Mediterranean, also won a FiFi award in 1996. Armani's latest perfume is Emporio Armani, described as a delicate oriental.

L'ARTISAN PARFUMEUR

A range of fragrances sold under a series of natural themes

PARENT COMPANY	*independent*
HEADQUARTERS	*Paris, France*
CURRENT PERFUMES	*Premier Figuier, Mûre et Musc, Mûre et Musc Extrême, Thé pour un Été, L'Eau de L'Artisan, L'Eau d'Ambre, Mimosa pour Moi, Drôle de Rose, Vanilla, and many others*

This is a small, exclusive perfume house founded in Paris by Jean Laporte in 1974. It is now run independently from him, but continues to sell some of his earlier fragrances as well as its own creations, using top-quality materials. It has its own exquisite boutiques in Paris and London, and outlets all over the world.

Besides providing around 25 high-quality fragrances for women, some at up to *eau de parfum* concentration, and others for men, it also sells room fragrances, scented candles, burning oils, sachets, and more. L'Artisan Parfumeur's fragrances are now sold under a series of natural olfactory themes: the Blackberry theme, for example, provides Mûre et Musc as an *eau de toilette*, Mûre et Musc Extrême as an *eau de parfum*, and Mûre Sauvage as a room fragrance; the very original Fig Tree line contains the top-selling *eau de toilette* Premier Figuier and a room fragrance called Intérieur Figuier; and in the same way the garden flower line includes six *eaux de toilette* products.

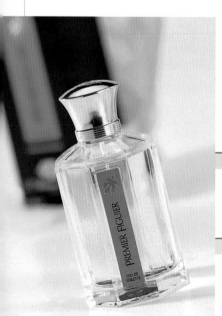

Premier Figuier

LAUNCHED	*1994*
CREATOR	*Olivia Jacobetti*
CATEGORY	*woody green*
FLACON	*standard "house" flacon*

notes

TOP	*fig leaves, galbanum*
MIDDLE	*almond milk, fig, sandalwood*
LOWER	*parasol lime, coconut, dried fruit*

BACCARAT

A fragrance that celebrates starry nights in India of old

PARENT COMPANY	*Taittinger*
HEADQUARTERS	*Paris, France*
CURRENT PERFUMES	*Une Nuit Étoilée au Bengale*

Two names head the list as makers of perfume bottles of the very highest quality—Baccarat and Lalique. Baccarat first started manufacturing lead crystal ware in the village of Baccarat, in Lorraine, France, in 1817. It produced its first perfume bottles soon after and has since supplied crystal flacons to almost all the leading perfume houses. Early Baccarat bottles can fetch huge prices at auction.

Recently Baccarat, which now belongs to the wealthy champagne family Taittinger, decided to enter the perfume market with a series of three limited-edition perfumes over a period of three years. Its first was Une Nuit Étoilée au Bengale (A Starry Night in Bengal). This is a sumptuous regardless-of-cost fragrance celebrating the days of the maharajahs in India (who had bought a lot of crystal ware in their time). The flacon, limited to 1,500 copies, is an elaborate design featuring a star-spangled arch containing a heart-shaped bottle in a presentation box.

Une Nuit Étoilée au Bengale

LAUNCHED	*1997*
CREATOR	*Christine Nagel (Quest)*
CATEGORY	*floral oriental amber*
FLACON	*Frederico Restrepo with Baccarat*

notes

TOP	*bergamot, rose*
MIDDLE	*sandalwood, Ceylonese spices, ginger, cinnamon*
LOWER	*amber, vanilla*

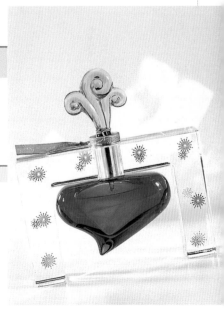

PARFUMS BALENCIAGA

Exquisite scents—the legacy of a leading fashion designer

PARENT COMPANY	*James Bogart since 1986*
HEADQUARTERS	*Paris, France*
CURRENT PERFUMES	*Le Dix, Quadrille, Michelle, Prelude, Rumba, Ho Hang, Talisman, Talisman Eau Transparente*

Cristobal Balenciaga was known as "the couturier of couturiers." As a small boy in Spain he was so interested in couture that he opened his first fashion house when he was only 16, in 1911. The Spanish Civil War forced him to move to Paris, France, and there, over 30 years, he became one of the world's leading fashion designers.

He once said, "A couturier must be an architect for design, a sculptor for shape, a painter for color, a musician for harmony, and a philosopher for temperament." He was all of these things. Coco Chanel described him as "the only couturier able to design, cut, assemble, and sew a dress together entirely by himself."

But he was also a strange personality, difficult to know, a dandy, a recluse. At the age of 74, when he decided to retire from the business, he closed all his fashion

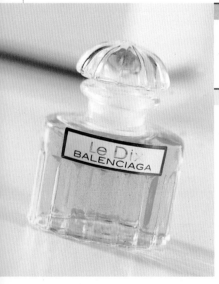

Le Dix

LAUNCHED	*1947*
CREATOR	*Roure perfumers*
CATEGORY	*floral woody aldehydic*
FLACON	*Bormidi*

notes

TOP	*bergamot, peach, lemon, cilantro*
MIDDLE	*rose, jasmine, orris, ylang-ylang, lily of the valley*
LOWER	*sandalwood, vetiver, civet, musk, vanilla*

Rumba

LAUNCHED *1988*
CREATOR *Givaudan perfumers*
CATEGORY *fruity floral*
FLACON *St Gobain*

notes

TOP *plum, peach, bergamot, basil*
MIDDLE *orchid, magnolia, gardenia, jasmine, tuberose, French marigold*
LOWER *amber, vanilla, plum, leather·*

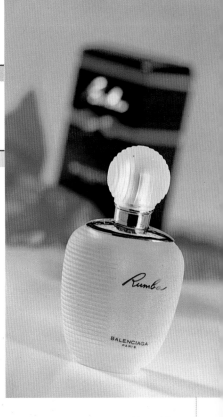

houses, in Paris, Barcelona, and Madrid and withdrew from the world until his death in 1972.

Fortunately, Balenciaga left an exquisite fragrance for posterity. He was well aware that the delicate notes of a scent were an essential adjunct to fashion design, and as soon as World War II was over he launched the classic perfume Le Dix. This was an immediate success, a scent evoking softness, beauty, and romanticism by a careful balance of floral and woody notes with aldehydes. It was named after the number of his house in the Avenue George V.

His next fragrance, Quadrille, followed some eight years later, a floral scent with fruity and spicy notes. But all subsequent perfumes date from after his retirement, when the tradition of producing scents of a very high quality was maintained. Notable among these is Rumba, launched in 1988, inspired by the energetic Latin-American dance and coming in a bottle modeled after a Roman vase. At present Balenciaga fragrances, like so many others, are made only at *eau de toilette* concentration—a great pity, but such are today's commercial restraints.

PARFUMS BALMAIN

The exclusive fashion house that has now become a worldwide business

PARENT COMPANY	*Laboroties Selecta Paris*
HEADQUARTERS	*Paris, France*
CURRENT PERFUMES	*Vent Vert, Jolie Madame, Miss Balmain, Ivoire, Balmain de Balmain*

Pierre Balmain (1914–83) believed in the importance of perfume in fashion long before he set up his own distinguished fashion house in Paris, France, in 1945. Almost concurrently he founded Parfums Balmain and launched a remarkably innovative new perfume, Vent Vert. He also believed in the advantages of high-quality art in advertising and employed for that purpose the leading French commercial illustrator of the day, René Gruau, well known for his brilliant designs promoting the perfumes of Dior.

Vent Vert was to become a classic fragrance. So, too, was Balmain's next perfume, the highly successful chypre fragrance Jolie Madame, which was introduced in 1953. Since those early days Balmain's exclusive fashion house has become a worldwide business selling a large variety of products for

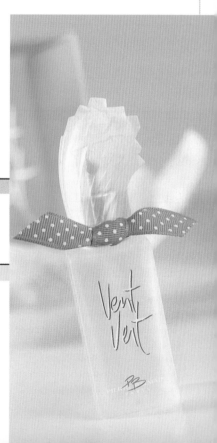

Vent Vert

LAUNCHED	*1945*
CREATOR	*Germaine Cellier*
CATEGORY	*green floral*
FLACON	*n/a*

notes

TOP	*galbanum*
MIDDLE	*rose, hyacinth, jasmine, lily of the valley*
LOWER	*oak moss, sage, sandalwood, musk*

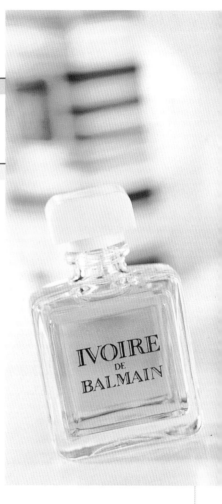

Ivoire

LAUNCHED *1979*
CREATOR *Florasynth perfumers*
CATEGORY *floral woody fruity*
FLACON *n/a*

notes

TOP *marigold, bergamot, galbanum, wormwood, camomile*

MIDDLE *jasmine, lily of the valley, rose, orris, jonquil, neroli*

LOWER *frankincense, vetiver, sandalwood, amber*

men and women looking for good taste and high quality.

Vent Vert was created by Germaine Cellier, one of the few women "noses" of the time, who worked for the prominent fragrance manufacturer Roure (now Givaudan-Roure). It is distinguished as the first of the so-called green perfumes, no other fragrance of this type being marketed for another 18 years. However, when the company relaunched it in 1991, they decided to change the formula, by adding floral notes, to suit modern taste.

Ivoire is a high-quality creation composed around some interesting ingredients by a team from the former American fragrance manufacturers Florasynth (now a part of Haarman & Reimer). It comes in a square-shaped flacon sealed inside a mock-ivory covering. Balmain's latest perfume, Balmain de Balmain was released in 1998.

BIJAN

The house that produced one of the strongest and most expensive perfumes on the market

PARENT COMPANY	*independent*
HEADQUARTERS	*New York, USA*
CURRENT PERFUMES	*Bijan Perfume for Women, DNA*

DNA

LAUNCHED *1993*
CREATOR *Claude Dir (Mane)*
CATEGORY *floral amber*
FLACON *Bijan Pakzad*

notes

TOP *rosewood, bergamot, geranium, ylang-ylang*
MIDDLE *jasmine, muguet, tuberose, osmanthus, clove*
LOWER *myrrh, oak moss, sandalwood, vetiver, vanilla, benzoin*

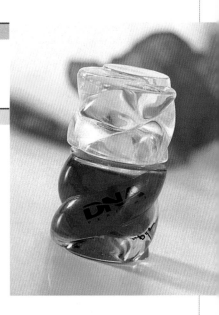

This is the perfume house of Bijan Pakzad, the American designer of Persian origin who set up what was at first a fashion company for men in Hollywood in 1976. His boutique in Rodeo Drive, Beverly Hills, soon became a favorite place for top film stars.

After producing a men's fragrance (in a crystal flacon by Baccarat) in 1981, he launched Bijan Perfume for Women in 1987, a floral-oriental fragrance created for him by Peter Bohm and sold in a high-quality ring-shaped flacon; at the time it was one of the strongest and most expensive perfumes on the market.

Six years later came the award-winning DNA, the initial letters of the names of Pakzad's three children. The highly original bottle is pillar-shaped in a double-helix design (reflecting the shape of the DNA molecule found in chromosomes). In 1997 the company also formed a new subsidiary through which it has launched Michael Jordan Cologne in conjunction with the basketball superstar of that name.

BOUCHERON

The jewelry house that sells a widely acclaimed perfume—in a jewel

PARENT COMPANY	*Parfums et Cosmétiques Internationales*
HEADQUARTERS	*Paris, France*
CURRENT PERFUMES	*Boucheron, Jaipur*

The family business of Boucheron have been making and selling top-quality jewelry ever since 1858. They catered for royals and the very rich, once even being chosen to estimate the value of the Persian crown jewels. Their products included perfume bottles for elegant boudoirs, so it was in keeping when Alain Boucheron decided to introduce a luxurious perfume.

"Noses" from the great Swiss perfume makers, Firmenich, composed the fragrance, using strongly contrasting notes and the very best of materials. A jewel-like flacon, resembling a giant Boucheron ring with a cabochon stopper, was designed. The new perfume was launched in 1988 and was widely acclaimed. Six years later Jaipur followed, created by IFF's leading perfumer, Sophia Grosjman, to invoke memories of the romantic fragrances of India. Both are perfumes of the highest quality.

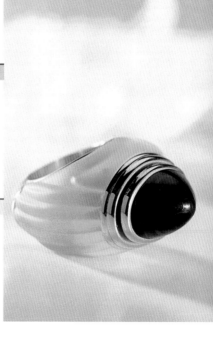

Boucheron

LAUNCHED	*1988*
CREATORS	*Francis Deléamont and Jean-Pierre Béthouart (Firmenich)*
CATEGORY	*floral semi-oriental*
FLACON	*Joël Desgrippes in association with Alain Boucheron*

notes

TOP	*tangerine, bitter orange, galbanum, tagetes, basil, apricot*
MIDDLE	*broom, ylang-ylang, tuberose, jasmine, orange flower, narcissus*
LOWER	*sandalwood, amber, tonka, vanilla*

BOURJOIS

The house that once boasted "the most famous fragrance in the world"

PARENT COMPANY	*Chanel*
HEADQUARTERS	*Paris, France*
CURRENT PERFUMES	*Soir de Paris, Mon Parfum, Évasion, Flamme, Stephanie*

The main business of Bourjois has always been make-up, but in its time it has produced some distinguished perfumes. Founded by Alexandre-Napoleon Bourjois in Paris, France, in 1863, the company sold theatrical make-up and face powders, but its cosmetic creations were soon extended to the Parisiennes (using the famous mark "Fabrique Spéciale pour la Beauté des Dames") and a large factory was built at Pantin. Bourjois made the first dry rouge and the first powder compact and started to produce fragrances in 1900, many in bottles by Baccarat. Their best seller was created by Ernest Beaux, of Chanel No5 fame, with the trend-setting Evening in Paris (later Soir de Paris), once called "the most famous fragrance in the world." In 1992 this classic perfume was re-formulated by Chanel's leading perfumers and is now sold in a brilliantly inexpensive edition at *eau de parfum* concentration in a midnight-blue, half-moon-shaped bottle.

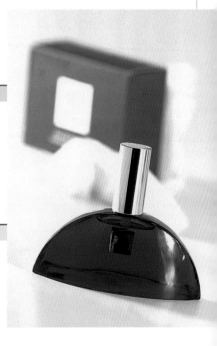

Soir de Paris

LAUNCHED	*1929, relaunched 1992*
CREATOR	*Ernest Beaux (reformulated in 1992 by Jacques Polge and François Demachy of Chanel)*
CATEGORY	*sweet floral*
FLACON	*Jean Helleu*

notes

TOP	*violet, fruity notes*
MIDDLE	*tilleul, clover, lilac, rose, jasmine*
LOWER	*vetiver, styrax, cedar, vanilla*

BVLGARI PARFUMS

Fragrances with an unusual and very distinctive signature

PARENT COMPANY	*independent*
HEADQUARTERS	*Neuchâtel, Switzerland*
CURRENT PERFUMES	*Bvlgari pour Femme, Eau Parfumée, Eau Parfumée Extrême, Cologne au Thé Vert*

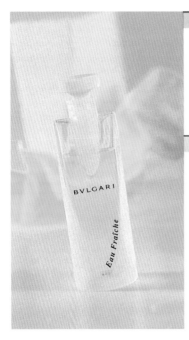

Bvlgari pour Femme

LAUNCHED	*1984 (reformulated 1993)*
CREATOR	*Jean-Claude Ellena (Givaudan-Roure): reformulation by Sophia Grosjman (IFF)*
CATEGORY	*green floral*
FLACON	*Thierry de Baschmakoff*

notes

TOP	*rosewood, ylang-ylang, hesperides, tea*
MIDDLE	*jasmine, violet, mimosa, rose, tea*
LOWER	*iris, vetiver, musk*

Bvlgari became famous as a family watch and jewelry business, but it has now made a very successful entry into the world of perfume. The Bvlgari family, originally Greek silversmiths, headed for Rome in the 1880s and opened a jewelry store. They prospered and have now become the world's largest jewelers after Cartier and Tiffany, with over 60 prestigious stores. Bvlgari Parfums was established in 1992 in Neuchâtel, Switzerland, as a separate division of the holding company (see Ferregamo page 91).

All their fragrances have an unusual and distinctive signature: they carry a green-tea note, around which the fragrance is constructed. Bvlgari pour Femme was the first launch in 1984, and is sold in *eau de parfum* concentration. After the company had set up Bvlgari Parfums as an independent division in 1992, this perfume was reformulated by the noted perfumer Sophia Grosjman and a fresher, less concentrated version called Eau Fraîche was added to the range.

PARFUMS CACHAREL

Makers of Anaïs-Anaïs—so good they say it twice

PARENT COMPANY	*L'Oréal*
HEADQUARTERS	*Paris, France*
CURRENT PERFUMES	*Anaïs-Anaïs, Loulou, Eau d'Eden, Noa*

Jean Bousquet comes from Provence and when he opened his fashion house in Paris, France, in 1962 he called it by the name of a small wild duck found in the Provençal countryside. Bousquet made his name as a leader in ready-to-wear fashion. Seventeen years later he appeared in the world of perfume with what has turned out to be a tireless bestseller, Anaïs-Anaïs, launched by Parfums Cacharel in 1979.

The inspiration for Anaïs-Anaïs came in fact from L'Oréal, who wanted to market a fragrance that would fit into the new ready-to-wear fashion image and could be sold inexpensively. Parfums Cacharel fitted their need as the right perfume house for this enterprise.

The project started, as so often happens in making a new fragrance, with the name. Anaïs derived from Anaïtis, an ancient Persian, and later Greek, goddess of life and death, but doubling it to Anaïs-Anaïs achieved a better sound. The notes of the new

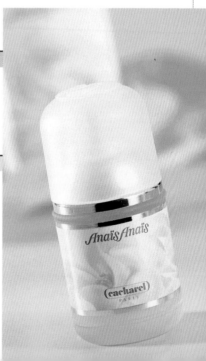

Anaïs-Anaïs

LAUNCHED	*1979*
CREATOR	*Roger Pellegrino and others (Firmenich)*
CATEGORY	*floral*
FLACON	*Annegret Beier*

notes

TOP	*orange blossom, lavender, lemon, hyacinth*
MIDDLE	*tuberose, jasmine, honeysuckle, lily of the valley, rose, carnation, iris, ylang-ylang*
LOWER	*sandalwood, cedar, vetiver, amber, incense, musk, leather, oak moss, patchouli*

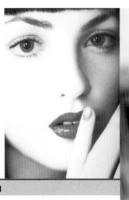

Loulou

LAUNCHED *1987*
CREATOR *Jean Guichard*
(Givaudan-Roure)
CATEGORY *floral oriental*
FLACON *Annegret Beier*

notes

TOP *jasmine, orange blossom, mimosa, lily, iris, cassie, ylang-ylang*
MIDDLE *heliotrope, iris*
LOWER *tonka, vanilla, frankincense, sandalwood*

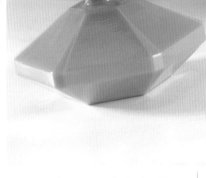

perfume were to be fresh, tender, and romantic, to attract a young clientele; to achieve this a group of Firmenich perfumers built up the fragrance around the lily and a range of highly scented white flowers, the first time this had been done.

TOP LEFT: *Advertisement for Loulou Blue.*

The bottle followed, designed by Annegret Beier, who has designed all the Cacharel bottles; she made it in white opaline, an innovation, with a silver cap and a label design of imaginary flowers. Anaïs-Anaïs was altogether new and has been one of the biggest-selling perfumes of all time.

Parfums Cacharel has subsequently launched Loulou, Eden, Loulou Blue, and Eau d'Eden, though not all are still being marketed. Loulou, a floral oriental fragrance, was named after the seductive yet innocent heroine played by the film star Louise Brooks in the 1929 film *Pandora's Box*, and is produced in a blue opaline bottle with a red cap, inspired by art deco designs of the 1920s and 30s. Noa was launched at the end of 1998 in the United States.

PARFUMS CARON

The perfume house with a greater range of labels than any other

PARENT COMPANY	*Caron-Révillon*
HEADQUARTERS	*Paris, France*
CURRENT PERFUMES	*Narcisse Noir, Infini, Nuit de Noël, Bellodgia, Fleur de Rocaille, Parfum Sacré and many others*

At the start of the twentieth century, in the Rue Rossini in Paris, a tiny perfumery and haberdashery store called Magasin Caron was purchased by a young perfumer, Ernest Daltroff. He liked the name and decided to retain it for his own business. Thus emerged Parfums Caron.

In 1906 Daltroff created an acclaimed perfume called Chantecler, which he sold in a flacon designed by Félicie Vanpouille. She became his business partner, designed most of his later flacons and, although she never married him, was his lover and eventually his heir.

In 1911 they launched Narcisse Noir and, in 1912, Infini, both to become huge successes, especially in the USA, where Daltroff and his contemporary Coty soon epitomized "French perfumes." Many new perfumes followed. Among them, Fleur de Rocaille, a famous floral perfume, evokes the fullness and vibrancy of spring as an Impressionist painter might have conceived it. It has been described as Daltroff's masterpiece.

Daltroff died in 1940 and Félicie married and continued running the business until her retirement in 1962. The company, now sells its fragrances widely and has a greater range of labels than any other perfume house. Its latest fragrance, Aimez Moi, was launched in 1997.

Fleur de Rocaille

LAUNCHED	*1933*
CREATOR	*Ernest Daltroff*
CATEGORY	*floral*
FLACON	*Félicie Vanpouille, later Michel Morsetti and Joël Desgrippes*

notes

TOP	*rosewood, bergamot*
MIDDLE	*jasmine, carnation, rose, orris, jonquil*
LOWER	*sandalwood, musk,*

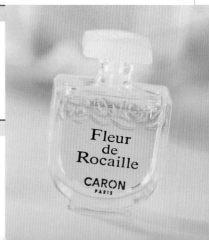

CARTIER

By royal appointment—the international company famous for more than just perfume

PARENT COMPANY	*Vendôme*
HEADQUARTERS	*Paris, France*
CURRENT PERFUMES	*Must de Cartier, Panthère, Must de Cartier II, So Pretty, Must de Cartier EdT, Déclaration*

Must de Cartier

LAUNCHED	*1981*
CREATOR	*Jean-Jacques Diener (Givaudan)*
CATEGORY	*oriental*
FLACON	*Xavier Rousseau and in-house*

notes

TOP	*galbanum, mandarin, neroli*
MIDDLE	*rose, daffodil, jasmine*
LOWER	*vanilla, sandalwood, vetiver, musk, tonka, civet*

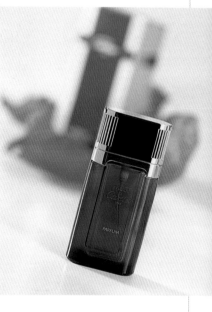

King Edward VII of England, when Prince of Wales, described Cartier as "jeweler of kings and king of jewelers." Such was the reputation of this great company at the turn of the century, built up since Jean-François Cartier (1819–1904) founded it in 1847. Before the 1850s were over Princess Eugénie was one of his clients.

Not long after Cartier's death the company held royal warrants from the monarchs of England, Spain, Portugal, Greece, Serbia, Belgium, Romania, Egypt, Siam, and Russia. Jewelry bracelet watches were first made by Cartier in 1888. In 1902 the Cartier workshops had orders for 27 jeweled diadems for women attending King Edward's coronation.

In 1910 Pierre Cartier bought the famous blue "Hope" diamond to resell. In 1917 he exchanged a double-row pearl necklace for the mansion in Fifth Avenue that was to become Cartier's American headquarters. In 1969 queues formed outside that mansion to see the famous diamond that Cartier had sold on

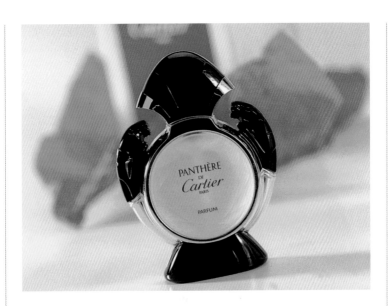

Panthère

LAUNCHED *1987*
CREATOR *Firmenich perfumers*
CATEGORY *floral woody*
FLACON *in-house*

notes

TOP *tuberose, orange flower, rose, jasmine, mandarin, labdanum*

MIDDLE *iris, sandalwood, vetiver, patchouli, nutmeg, oak moss*

LOWER *civet, musk, ambergris, vanilla, opopanax*

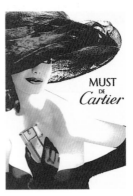

ABOVE: *Must de Cartier— luxurious simplicity.*

to Elizabeth Taylor for her birthday-gift necklace from Richard Burton. The history of Cartier contains many such events.

Under Louis Cartier, grandson of the founder, the company expanded worldwide, but with his death in 1942 and other problems it split into separately run units in Paris, London, and New York. These were not reunited until 1972, when Joseph Kanoui and a group of investors bought them up and appointed Robert Hocq as chairman. It was Hocq who created the concept of Le Must de Cartier (simply an article that someone must have) and launched the opening all over the world of Must de Cartier boutiques.

When Hocq died in a car accident in 1973 Kanoui himself took over. The company became a part of the Vendôme group (along with other luxury companies like Montblanc, Dunhill, Karl Lagerfeld, and Chloé) in 1993. Perfume came late into the Cartier inventories with the launch of the oriental Must de Cartier in 1981. This was an important perfume, originating from the notion of having a fragrance for evening wear which could be worn over the top of one for day wear. A creation by Jean-Jacques Diener of Givaudan-Roure was chosen for the evening one and launched, as Must de Cartier, in a bottle designed in-house by Xavier Rousseau to replicate the refillable gold-plated cigarette lighter Cartier was selling.

The daytime perfume never materialized. The floral-woody perfume Panthère, of 1987, followed the launching of the company's Panthère watch, with a beautiful flacon depicting stylized panthers. Must de Cartier II, a high-quality floral perfume created by Alberto Morillas of Firmenich, came out in 1993. Two years later Cartier launched So Pretty, an award-winning *eau de parfum* in a bottle designed with the help of Joël Desgrippes and which features Cartier's well-known three-ring symbol; this launch commemorated the wedding of Louis Cartier a century before to the granddaughter of Charles Worth, the couturier, for he called her "My So Pretty." More recently Cartier have launched Must de Cartier Eau de Toilette, which is a new version of the original Must fragrance, and Déclaration, which was produced as a men's fragrance but has proved to be a remarkably popular scent with women as well.

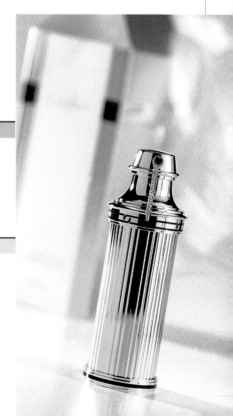

So Pretty

LAUNCHED *1995*

CREATOR *Jean Guichard (Givaudan-Roure)*

CATEGORY *floral*

FLACON *Joël Desgrippes and in-house*

notes

TOP *mandarin, neroli, bergamot, dewberry, jasmine*

MIDDLE *rose, iris, peach, osmanthus, diamond orchid*

LOWER *vetiver, oak moss, benzoin, sandalwood*

CARVEN PARFUMS

Maker of Ma Griffe, the perfume that fell from the sky....

PARENT COMPANY	*International Classic Brands*
HEADQUARTERS	*London, England*
CURRENT PERFUMES	*Ma Griffe, Intrigue, Madame Guirlandes, Eau Vive*

In 1945, immediately after World War II had ended, a new couture house for the petite was opened in Paris, France, by Mademoiselle Carven, whose real name was Carmen de Tomaso. She had the support of three businessmen friends who had been prisoners of war together. Little time was lost in organizing a perfume to go with the clothes Mlle Carven was designing; the top "nose" at Roure was engaged and in 1946 Ma Griffe was introduced.

The launch was sensational: thousands of miniature bottles of the new perfume were dropped over Paris by tiny green and white parachutes. Ma Griffe broke new ground with the use of a newly discovered synthetic obtained from gardenia, which added a dry sharpness to the fragrance. It was the first perfume created especially for the younger woman, teenagers, and debutantes, and used the slogan "Ma Griffe—le parfum jeune" (a "griffe" is a silk label and the name signified "It's mine").

Carven was also the first perfume house to sponsor sporting

Ma Griffe

LAUNCHED	*1946*
CREATOR	*Jean Carles*
CATEGORY	*green mossy floral*
FLACON	*Pochet et du Courval*

notes

TOP	*gardenia, citrus, galbanum, aldehydes*
MIDDLE	*jasmine, lily of the valley, rose, ylang-ylang, iris*
LOWER	*styrax, oak moss, sandalwood, cinnamon, benzoin, labdanum, musk, vetiver*

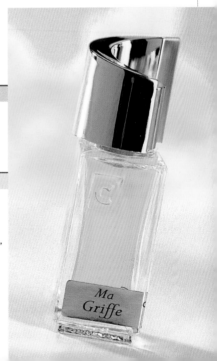

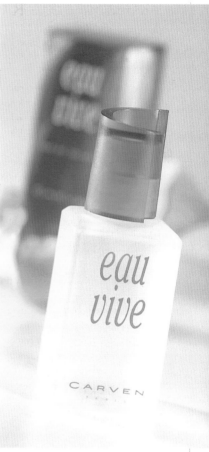

Eau Vive

LAUNCHED	*1996 (another perfume of this name launched by Carven in 1966)*
CREATOR	*Quest perfumers*
CATEGORY	*citrus aromatic*
FLACON	*standard bottle*

notes

TOP	*green citrus*
MIDDLE	*fennel, cilantro, juniper, mandarin, lavender*
LOWER	*musk, vanilla*

events of the more elegant type (yachting, tennis, horse riding), the first to sell its perfumes on airlines, the first to offer literary awards to young writers. But, despite launching other famous perfumes such as Madame de Carven and Intrigue, things went wrong: the company had to cut back and eventually distribution rights were bought up by Shulton, the manufacturers of Old Spice, who did not make a success of them. Carven Parfums was then bought by an Englishman, David Reiner, who, through his company International Classic Brands, also owned Worth. He has launched new fragrances—Madame Guirlandes (a development from the amalgamation of Madame de Carven and Guirlandes) and Eau Vive (an *eau fraîche* for summer months)—and retained others. In 1998 he announced that he was putting both Carven and Worth up for sale.

PARFUMS CERRUTI

The worldwide fashion empire with fragrances for both men and women

PARENT COMPANY	*Parfums International/Elizabeth Arden*
HEADQUARTERS	*Paris, France*
CURRENT PERFUME	*Cerruti 1881 pour Femme*

The firm of Nino Cerruti was founded in 1881, which is why that date is included in the name of its latest perfume. The founders were three Cerruti brothers who lived in Italy and started up a business to produce woolen materials and, in due course, other textiles (so there is also a textile theme in their perfume).

The present head of the firm, Nino Cerruti, born in 1930 and a grandson of one of the founders, has developed the business into a worldwide fashion empire with its headquarters in Paris, France. But the fragrance division, Parfums Cerruti, was bought in 1987 by Elizabeth Arden, who have themselves since been acquired by Unilever, and who run it through their subsidiary, Parfums International.

The first Cerruti fragrance was for men and was launched in 1979; a corresponding perfume for women issued later is no longer on the market and the only women's perfume they now sell is Cerruti 1881 pour Femme, a fragrance of high quality which they launched, at *parfum* concentration, in 1995. As a special side effect this uses an accord of aldehyde, freesia, and muguet, which is called Fleur de Lin and conveys a trace of the smell of linen.

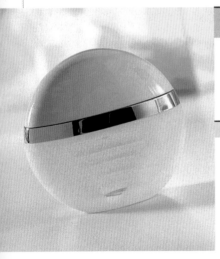

Cerruti 1881 pour Femme

LAUNCHED	*1995*
CREATOR	*Claire Cain (Givaudan-Roure)*
CATEGORY	*floral woody*
FLACON	*n/a*

notes

TOP	*mimosa, freesia, violet, bergamot, Fleur de Lin*
MIDDLE	*orange blossom, camomile, geranium, jasmine, rosewood, Fleur de Lin*
LOWER	*cedar, amber, musk, sandalwood*

CHANEL

A name known the world over—a fragrance sold by numbers

PARENT COMPANY	*Wertzheimer family*
HEADQUARTERS	*Paris, France*
CURRENT PERFUMES	*Chanel No5, Chanel No19, Chanel No22, Cristalle, Coco, Allure, Gardenia, Bois des Îles, Cuir de Russie*

There is no more famous perfume than Chanel No5, which Marilyn Monroe famously confessed was all she wore in bed, and no more legendary person in the world of fashion and perfume than Coco Chanel, who in 1921 selected it from five samples given to her by its creator, Ernest Beaux. She kept the number because it was her lucky number: her collections were always shown on the fifth day of the fifth month.

Coco Chanel was born in 1883, although very little is known about her early years. She opened a hat boutique in Paris in 1913, turned to couture, and took a leading part in the move away from the stiff fashion styles of the time. She produced the Total Look, with its complementary accessories, and then later the "little black dress." By 1935 she was employing over 2,000 seamstresses.

Odd as it may seem, for most of her life Coco Chanel did not own

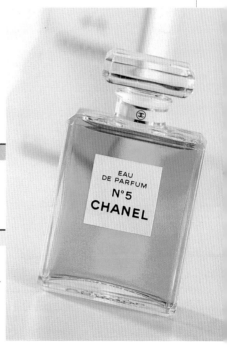

Chanel No5

LAUNCHED	*1921*
CREATOR	*Ernest Beaux*
CATEGORY	*floral aldehyde*
FLACON	*Coco Chanel*

notes

TOP	*ylang-ylang, neroli, aldehydes*
MIDDLE	*jasmine, rose, iris, lily of the valley*
LOWER	*sandalwood, vetiver, musk, vanilla, civet, oak moss*

Chanel No19

LAUNCHED	*1970*
CREATOR	*Henri Robert*
CATEGORY	*floral woody chypre*
FLACON	*derived from original design for No5*

notes

TOP	*galbanum*
MIDDLE	*neroli, orris, leather*
LOWER	*cedar, oak moss*

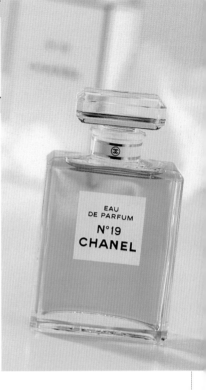

the perfume company that bore her name. To exploit the phenomenal success of No5 she needed finance, which she obtained from Pierre Wertheimer, a prominent business-man of that time. She launched several new fragrances over the decade up to 1931, including Chanel No22, Gardenia, Bois des Îles, and Cuir de Russie, but then, because of the war, and the closure of her fashion business, there was nothing more for 40 years. Chanel No19, the creation of Beaux's successor Henri Robert, was launched on 19 August, 1970, Chanel's 87th birthday. A few months later, she died.

Cristalle, in 1974, demonstrated Henri Robert's sure touch but it was an isolated venture. It was not until 1984 that interest in the house was revived, with the appointment of Karl Lagerfeld, and the creation of "Coco" by the new Chanel "nose," Jacques Polge.

In 1996 an innovative new perfume, Allure, was launched using a fragrance structure different from the usual three-tier one; it is described as having many facets with no one note predominating.

Chanel makes all its own fragrances, with their "nose," Jacques Polge and it retains special links with jasmine and May rose growers in Grasse to ensure it gets jasmine of an exceptionally high quality. The packaging for all fragrances is derived from the simple design originally chosen for No5 by Coco Chanel. The main Chanel perfume installations are now at Compiègne.

Ownership of Chanel remains with the Wertheimer family. For many years Chanel used a number of famous faces to advertise No5, including Catherine Deneuve (in the United States), and most recently Carole Bouquet, who is seen to represent the ideal Frenchwoman of today.

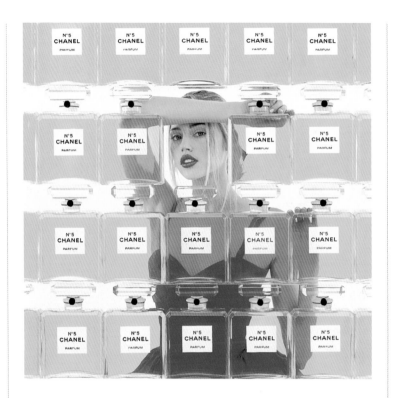

ABOVE: *The most famous fragrance in the world.*

Allure

LAUNCHED *1996*
CREATOR *Jacques Polge*
CATEGORY *abstract floral*
FLACON *derived from original design for No5*

notes

LINEAR *"fresh" from citrus, "fruity" from mandarin, "floral" from jasmine, "imaginary floral" from an accord of magnolia, honeysuckle, and waterlily, "woody" from vetiver, "oriental" from vanilla*

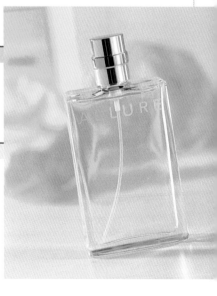

MARY CHESS

Opulent perfumes that are made from the very finest and most expensive natural ingredients

PARENT COMPANY	*Fine Fragrances and Cosmetics Group*
HEADQUARTERS	*London, England*
CURRENT PERFUME	*Tuberose*

Tuberose

LAUNCHED	*1937*
CREATOR	*Mary Chess*
CATEGORY	*single-note floral*
FLACON	*n/a*

notes

LINEAR	*Sweet, spicy floral based on tuberose*

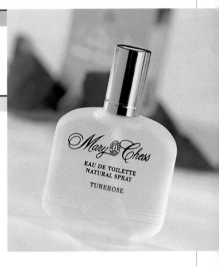

Mrs. Grace Mary Chess Robinson was an American from Kentucky who went to live in London during the 1920s. She loved flowers and herbs and became known for her beautiful "sculptured flowers," made from metal, clay, and parchment, which were purchased by, among others, Queen Mary. In 1932 she established the Mary Chess company, moving into a little store in Shepherd Market, in London's select Mayfair district, in 1948, and started to sell her own opulent perfumes, made by herself from the finest natural ingredients.

Her trademark was a chess queen, and the game of chess featured in many of her products. White Lilac was the first of her perfume creations and she must have felt enormous pride when it was once declared one of the eight great perfumes of the world.

In 1975 she was given a royal warrant as perfumer to the British Queen Mother. But the company lost its momentum and ceased to trade until, in 1991, it was acquired by Fine Fragrances and Cosmetics.

Two of the early perfumes, Autere and Tapestry, were relaunched in the early 1990s, but now the only perfume sold is the single-note *eau de toilette*, Tuberose, a classic rendition of one of the most highly esteemed fragrances used in perfumery.

PARFUMS CHLOÉ

A feminine fragrance created to be worn by the true romantic

PARENT COMPANY	*Parfums International / Elizabeth Arden*
HEADQUARTERS	*Paris, France*
CURRENT PERFUMES	*Chloé, Narcisse*

The fashion house of Chloé was set up in Paris, France, in 1952. Founded by Jacques Lenoir and Gaby Ashgion, it produced innovative ready-to-wear clothes and accessories for the luxury end of the market, designing many of the fabrics it used. There are now Chloé boutiques all round the world.

However, perfume did not come into the Chloé thinking for another 20 years until, in 1975, the company's newly established perfume division, Parfums Chloé, launched their signature fragrance, simply called Chloé. The impetus for this was provided by their new designer, Karl Lagerfeld, who has always seen fragrance as an integral part of fashion.

The fragrance itself, at *extrait* concentration, had 178 ingredients, built around tuberose. The flacon for it, designed by Joe Messina, was spherical with a sculptured lily on the stopper, and immediately won a FiFi design award. The same theme is repeated in later bottles. The

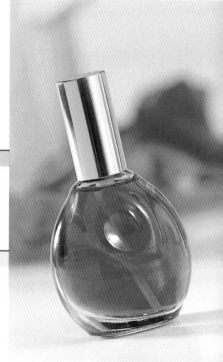

Chloé

LAUNCHED	*1975*
CREATOR	*IFF perfumers*
CATEGORY	*sweet floral*
FLACON	*Joe Messina (with Karl Lagerfeld)*

notes

TOP	*honeysuckle, orange flower, ylang-ylang, hyacinth*
MIDDLE	*jasmine, rose, narcissus, carnation, tuberose*
LOWER	*sandalwood, amber, oak moss, musk*

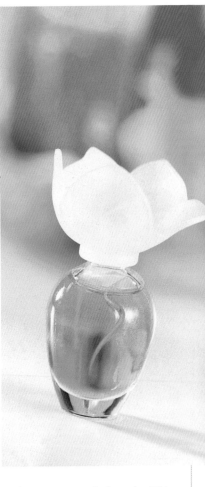

Narcisse

LAUNCHED *1992*
CREATOR *IFF perfumers*
CATEGORY *floral oriental*
FLACON *n/a*

notes

TOP *apricot, marigold, orange flower, plumiera*

MIDDLE *narcissus, rose, jasmine, spices*

LOWER *sandalwood, vanilla, musk, balsam of tolu*

fragrance has been described as feminine without being frivolous, to be worn by the true romantic.

The perfume Chloé was followed a few years later by Narcisse, a haunting fragrance created for the company by IFF perfumers with a heart that stresses the scent of narcissus. In the ancient legend, Narcissus was the boy who fell in love with his reflection in a pool, disappearing to be replaced by the flower. With a scent of mixed jasmine and hyacinth, narcissus has been used as an ingredient in perfumery since the earliest days.

In 1997 Chloé came up with a new green-powdery perfume called Innocence, made for the younger woman; it was not a success and has already been discontinued. Parfums Chloé now belongs to Unilever, who hold it as a part of Parfums International, which is administered by Elizabeth Arden.

CHOPARD

Creator of Wish, an innovative perfume with qualities that sparkle and glow

PARENT COMPANY	*Lancaster / Coty*
HEADQUARTERS	*Paris, France*
CURRENT PERFUMES	*Casmir, Wish*

The House of Chopard is one of Geneva's leading companies in the luxury watch and jewelry world. Founded as watchmakers in 1860, the firm added jewelry in 1963, when Paul André Chopard and Karl Scheufele amalgamated their two businesses. In 1994 they decided to extend their activities into perfumery and launched the very successful, innovative, prizewinning fruity-oriental perfume Casmir. It was created for them by Michel Almairac, the owner of Créations Aromatiques, and appeared in a lotus-shaped bottle designed by Chopard's own Caroline Scheufele.

After Heaven, an innovative fragrance for men brought out in 1995, they produced their second women's perfume two years later with Wish, which featured the diamond. This again is an innovative perfume of high quality, with some unusual notes to underline the theme (the "sparkle" of acacia, the "glow" of Chinese gooseberry, for example), composed by one of IFF's top perfumers.

The flacon resembles a multi-faceted cut diamond and comes in a midnight-blue case. The perfume house of Chopard belongs to the Lancaster Group, itself, since recently, a part of Coty.

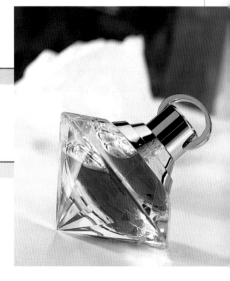

Wish

LAUNCHED	*1997*
CREATOR	*Nathalie Lorson (IFF)*
CATEGORY	*woody gourmet floral oriental*
FLACON	*Fabrice Legros*

notes

TOP	*acacia, honeysuckle, Chinese gooseberry*
MIDDLE	*osmanthus, patchouli, violet*
LOWER	*incense, amber, sandalwood*

CLARINS

Creator of a best-selling perfume that's a skin tonic as well as a feel-good fragrance

PARENT COMPANY	*independent*
HEADQUARTERS	*Neuilly-sur-Seine, France*
CURRENT PERFUME	*Eau Dynamisante*

Eau Dynamisante

LAUNCHED	*1987*
CREATOR	*Jacques Courtin-Clarins*
CATEGORY	*woody chypre*
FLACON	*Pierre Dinand*

notes

lemon, orange, cilantro, caraway, thyme, rosemary, patchouli

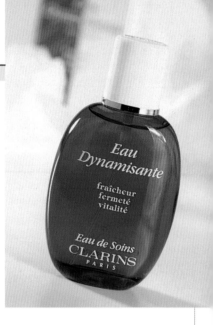

Clarins was founded in 1954 by a physiotherapist, Jacques Courtin-Clarins, who opened a beauty salon after noting the beneficial effects that his treatments using plant oils for massage were having on the skin. It has now become a very large cosmetics and fragrance company, particularly noted for its quality skin-care products and salons. Jacques Courtin-Clarins is still the president of the company, which has its headquarters and a major manufacturing complex at Neuilly-sur-Seine, near Paris, France.

In 1994 the company brought out its first perfume, Elysium, in an attractive bottle shaped to represent a river pebble with a leaf on its side, but this has recently been discontinued. Clarins's best-seller has always been Eau Dynamisante, first launched in 1987. This is a combined perfume and skin tonic, the first of such products, which is also now used by men and is described as a feel-good product.

But the company now has larger perfume interests, having acquired the Thierry Mugler, Azzaro, and Montana fragrances in 1995.

THE HOUSE OF COTY

The firm that began with a broken bottle and went on to conquer the world's market

PARENT COMPANY	*Benckiser*
HEADQUARTERS	*Paris, France*
CURRENT PERFUMES	*L'Aimant, Vanilla Fields, Monsoon, Exclamation, Chanson d'Eau, Quiditty, Monsoon Eau, Shimo, and others*

François Coty, a Corsican, regarded as "the father of modern perfumery," revolutionized the whole way in which the industry functioned and built an empire that dominated the perfume market for over 40 years. He learned his business in Grasse in southeast France and on his return to Paris set out to practice his own ideas about perfumes, making the most of newly invented synthetic materials and the latest technical advances.

Before the 1900s only the privileged rich had used scents; Coty wanted to seduce the emerging bourgeoisie. "Give a woman the best product you can make," he said "present it in a container of simple but impeccable taste, ask a reasonable price for it." That is still the Coty maxim. In 1904 he and his wife set up a laboratory and showroom for their scents in one room of their small Paris apartment.

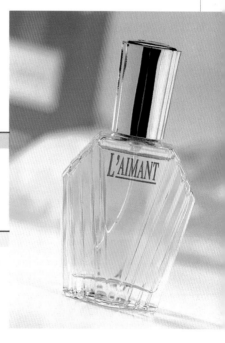

L'Aimant

LAUNCHED	*1927, relaunched 1995*
CREATOR	*François Coty and Vincent Roubert*
CATEGORY	*floral aldehyde*
FLACON	*n/a*

notes

TOP	*bergamot, neroli, peach, strawberry*
MIDDLE	*jasmine, rose, ylang-ylang*
LOWER	*vanilla, vetiver, sandalwood*

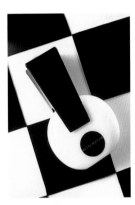

ABOVE: *Exclamation—launched in 1990.*

Coty took his first creation to the head buyer of the most prestigious department store in Paris, who refused to stock it. It is a well-known story that, on the way out, he let the bottle slip from his hand, so that the glass smashed and the fragrant aroma filled the store, starting an irresistable clamor for it from the store's customers.

In the following year he produced L'Origan, the first floral-oriental perfume and a huge success throughout the world. In the United States it was even made into a perfumed talc which sold by the million. From then on until his death in 1934 Coty produced over 50 perfumes. They included the first of the modern style of chypre perfume, which was simply called Chypre, and, in 1927, the famous L'Aimant fragrance, promoted as "the passionate woman's perfume," which took him some five years to perfect. Relaunched for a wide market in 1995, it is currently the best-selling fragrance in the United Kingdom.

Coty had an eye for beautifully designed bottles. Some 20 were made for him by Baccarat, but, more significantly, the store next to his own in the fashionable Place Vendôme was that of René Lalique, who became a close friend. Lalique provided 16 scent bottles for him, many being used for more than one perfume. They include some of the most elegant flacons ever made, eagerly sought after now by collectors.

Vanilla Fields

LAUNCHED	*1993*
CREATOR	*Fragrance Resources*
CATEGORY	*oriental vanilla*
FLACON	*in-house*

notes

vanilla, jasmine, mimosa

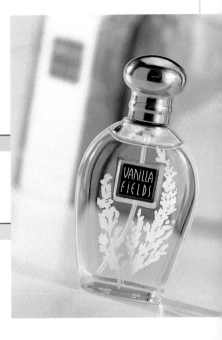

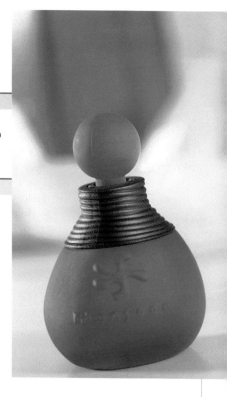

Monsoon

LAUNCHED *1994*
CREATOR *Maurice Roucel (Quest)*
CATEGORY *floral*
FLACON *Design in Action*

notes

TOP *lily, gardenia, ylang-ylang*
MIDDLE *green floral*
LOWER *amber, sandalwood, oak moss*

François Coty had become one of France's wealthiest men, been made a Senator in Corsica, assembled a fine collection of paintings and *objets d'art*, and obtained control of the newspaper *Le Figaro,* but there was no happy ending. A costly divorce and the 1929 Wall Street crash ruined him.

However, after his death new fragrances continued to appear, among them the innovative, prizewinning, and trend-setting Vanilla Fields, which was made for a wide market and became the number-one-selling fragrance in the whole of the United States. Monsoon, made in conjunction with the fashion house of that name, has also been highly successful and comes in an unusual aquamarine bottle with a conical copper-colored cap.

In 1992 the Coty company passed to Benckiser, who have reorganized it to tie it in with their other fragrance and cosmetic interests. Coty Inc. now has a Coty division, which looks after volume fragrances and cosmetics, and a Lancaster division, which handles the bulk of the prestige products, including designer fragrances such as Jil Sander and Joop! With its recent acquisition of Unilever's cosmetics businesses, Coty is now the largest marketer of mass fragrances in the world, an achievement of which François Coty would undoubtedly have been very proud.

THE HOUSE OF CREED

The family-owned perfume house that caters to the famous

PARENT COMPANY	*independent*
HEADQUARTERS	*Paris, France*
CURRENT PERFUMES	*Spring Flower, Fleurissimo, Fleurs de Bulgarie, Fantasia de Fleurs, Vanisia, Royal Delight, Jasmine Imperatrice Eugénie, Tubereuse Indiana, Jasmal, Royal Water, and others*

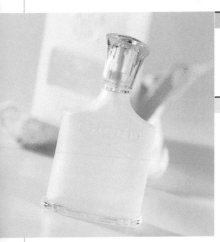

Royal Water

LAUNCHED	*1997*
CREATOR	*Oliver Creed*
CATEGORY	*fresh green*
FLACON	*Olivier Creed*

notes

TOP	*hesperides*
MIDDLE	*basil, mint, cumin, juniper, pepper*
LOWER	*musk, ambergris*

This is a small, family-owned perfume house providing very high-quality fragrances of *eau de parfum* strength from its factory near Fontainebleau in France. James Creed founded the company as a London tailoring business in 1760, but it really started as a perfumery in Paris in 1854, supplying many crowned heads and their courts, including Queen Victoria of England. Its present president, Oliver Creed, a direct descendant of James, is himself the firm's creative perfumer, and his fragrances, sometimes made exclusively for his clients, contain the highest percentage of natural components of any in the French perfume industry.

Over the years the company has produced more than 200 perfumes, its latest scent being Royal Water, an unusual fresh green aromatic fragrance with a hint of sexiness.

Many famous women have patronized Creed in recent times, including Grace Kelly (Prince Rainier commissioned Fleurissimo for her for their wedding), Jacqueline Onassis, Madonna, and Naomi Campbell.

CROWN PERFUMERY

Creator of high-class, single-note perfumes based on old formulas

PARENT COMPANY	*independent*
HEADQUARTERS	*London, England*
CURRENT PERFUMES	*Marechale, Marechale 90, Crown Stephanotis, Crown Bouquet, Malabar, Matsukita, Crown Court Bouquet*

The present Crown Perfumery, with a sophisticated little period store in London's fashionable Burlington Arcade in Mayfair, is a revival of what was once one of Britain's foremost perfume houses. It sells a wide range of its own high-quality, single-note scents.

The original business was founded in 1872 by an American-born maker of crinolines and corsets, William Sparks Thomson, and his two sons. They entered the market with a collection of floral scents called Flower Fairies and made their fortune with Crown Lavender Smelling Salts.

By the end of the century the company had built its own factory at St Katherine's docks and was exporting nearly 50 different fragrances and beauty products to countries all over the world, some in distinguished flacons by Baccarat. Crown invented the system of "perfume layering," now being revived, where one perfume is applied over the top of one already being worn in order to enrich it.

Marechale 90

LAUNCHED	*relaunched 1994*
CREATOR	*n/a*
CATEGORY	*floral chypre*
FLACON	*n/a*

notes

TOP	*bergamot, ylang-ylang, galbanum, basil*
MIDDLE	*rose, jasmine, muguet, orris, cloves, cardamom*
LOWER	*patchouli, cistus, amber, musk, herbal undertones*

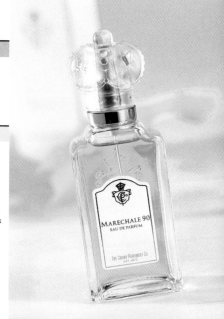

Thomson even invented a means of perfuming the air in the auditorium of London's Gaiety Theatre before performances. But after his death in the 1920s the company was sold to Lever Brothers, who converted the factory to making hair products and eventually, in 1939, closed it down.

The revival has been brought about by Barry Gibson, an industrial chemist related to the Thomson family, who acquired the archives and sought to re-create a new version of the original business. In 1994 Crown Perfumery was relaunched, selling 27 high-class, single-note

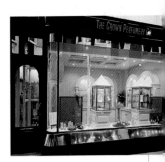

ABOVE: *Crown Perfumery's London store.*

perfumes, mostly based on the early original formulas and composed from natural materials.

Marechale, with more than 70 ingredients, is an impeccable floral scent devised from a formula of 1669 which was found in Crown Perfumery's archives. It was created for a distinguished client, Madame de Marechale d'Aumont, and is now their prestige perfume. It is a limited edition with only 250 bottles having been produced. However, the company have produced a contemporized version of this exclusive fragrance, Marechale 90. It is a floral-chypre perfume, with highlighted green notes. Crown Bouquet, one of the most successful scents produced by the original company, was at first called Crab Apple Blossom. It was designed, and is still used, for "perfume layering" over Matsukita for evening wear.

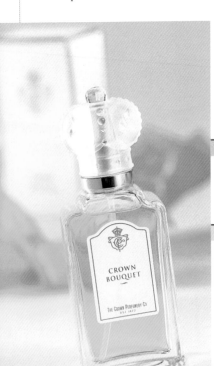

Crown Bouquet

LAUNCHED *relaunched 1994*
CREATOR *n/a*
CATEGORY *fresh green floral*
FLACON *n/a*

notes

include hyacinth, rose, jasmine, tuberose, gardenia

PARFUMS SALVADOR DALI

Fragrance and art—and the art of the perfumer—in startlingly original bottles

PARENT COMPANY	*COFCI*
HEADQUARTERS	*Paris, France*
CURRENT PERFUMES	*Le Parfum, Laguna, Dalissime, Eau de Dali, Dalimix (unisex), Le Roy Soleil, Dalimix Gold*

While working on one of his paintings, *Apparition du Visage l'Aphrodite de Cnide,* in 1981, the surrealist artist Salvador Dali was approached by a group of businessmen from the recently established French fragrance firm Compaignie Française de Commerce Internationale. They wondered whether he would be interested in working with them on a new fragrance concept. Dali was enthusiastic and used the canvas of his incomplete painting to illustrate his ideas about flacons with sketches which he then retained in the final painting.

From this meeting emerged Parfums Salvador Dali with a range, now, of 10 fragrances in startlingly original bottles. Le Parfum (also called Salvador Dali) was the first fragrance to be produced, launched in 1985 in a flacon portraying the nose and mouth of the Aphrodite in Dali's picture. The picture itself, for which he had used the famous statue by Praxiteles as his model, was reproduced on the packaging.

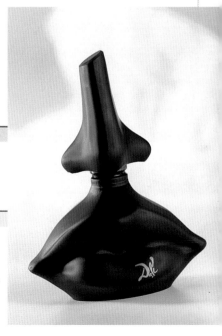

Le Parfum

LAUNCHED	*1985*
CREATOR	*Givaudan perfumers*
CATEGORY	*floral oriental*
FLACON	*Salvador Dali*

notes

TOP	*green, fruity*
MIDDLE	*rose, jasmine, orange-flower*
LOWER	*amber, cedarwood, musk, vanilla, myrrh*

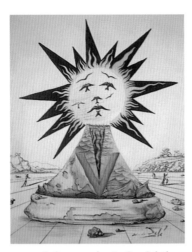

ABOVE: *Dali watercolor, Le Roy Soleil.*

The fragrance contained rose because of his wife Gala's beloved rose garden, and jasmine because he often wore a sprig of it behind his ear when he was painting. A men's fragrance showing the mouth and chin of Aphrodite followed, but was delayed because of Gala's death and Dali's subsequent breakdown.

Dali himself died in 1989 and, as a tribute, the company launched an *eau de toilette*, Laguna, in 1990.

In 1994 came Dalissime, a fruity-floral perfume created by Marc Buxton (Haarmann & Reimer) and was issued to commemorate the centennial of Gala's birthday. The bottle is shaped in the form of a Corinthian pillar in a nose-and-mouth shape which featured in a Dali painting called *Christmas*.

Dalimix (1966) is unisex and the flacon shows a man's chin below a woman's mouth. Lastly, in 1997, Le Roy Soleil was launched, in an eye-catching bottle similar to one Schiaparelli had used for her own perfume. Le Roy Soleil's flacon is taken from a Dali watercolor, painted to mark the end of World War II.

Le Roy Soleil

LAUNCHED	*1997*
CREATOR	*Phillipe Romano*
CATEGORY	*fruity oriental*
FLACON	*designed by Salvador Dali, made by Baccarat*

notes

TOP	*bergamot, lemon, pawpaw, pineapple, rosewood*
MIDDLE	*clove, cinnamon, cyclamen, rose, jasmine, apricot*
LOWER	*patchouli, sandalwood, vetiver, tonka, vanilla, musk*

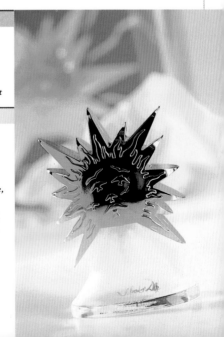

DAVIDOFF

A scent as refreshing as water, conveying the idea of crystal-clear mountain lakes

PARENT COMPANY	*Horst Geberding Holding*
HEADQUARTERS	*Geneva, Switzerland*
CURRENT PERFUMES	*Cool Water Woman, Good Life*

Davidoff is a brand name covering two fragrances, Cool Water (made for men) and Cool Water Woman. Cool Water was first marketed in 1988, heavily advertised (for example, over 11 million scent strips were inserted in magazines) and quickly became a best-seller. Cool Water Woman did not follow until 1997. It is sold as "a scent as refreshing as water itself" and aims to convey the idea of luminous, crystal-clear, cool bodies of water, like mountain lakes.

The mastermind behind this perfume is a distinguished perfumer, Pierre Bourdon, the creator, among others, of Dolce Vita for Dior. After working for Roure, Bourdon helped set up the European branch of the perfume creation firm Takasago, was then Director of Creation at Quest, and finally set up his own company Fragrance Resources. Cool Water Woman is made in a line up to *eau de toilette* concentration and appears in a translucent-blue flacon designed in the form of a drop of water.

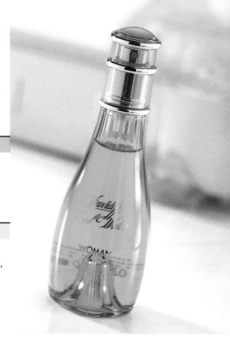

Cool Water Woman

LAUNCHED	*1997*
CREATOR	*Pierre Bourdon*
CATEGORY	*fresh aquatic*
FLACON	*Peter Schmidt*

notes

TOP	*citrus, quince, blackcurrant, pineapple, melon*
MIDDLE	*rose, jasmine, muguet, lotus, waterlily*
LOWER	*orris, vetiver, sandalwood*

DESPREZ

A firm that aimed for only the highest quality, creating products of good taste

PARENT COMPANY	*Parlux Fragrances*
HEADQUARTERS	*Paris, France*
CURRENT PERFUMES	*Bal à Versailles, Sheherazade*

Desprez is another of those many perfume houses that have found the economic blizzards of the 1990s hard to sail through. It is not an old firm, having been founded in 1938 by Jean Desprez, a professional perfumer (born 1898), who was a great-grandson of the well-known Felix Millot.

Millot had started his perfume work in the 1860s, in the days when his Bears Fat Pomade had great appeal, and the firm was eventually passed on to his other great-grandson, Henri Desprez. The two worked together in Paris, France, and Jean created the classic perfume Crêpe de Chine for Millot in 1925.

Jean Desprez wanted to sell only products of the very highest quality and good taste. He employed Leon Leyritz, a talented sculptor, to design the flacons and the artist Paul Mergier to design the packaging.

In 1939 three significant perfumes were launched: Votre Main, Grande Dame, in a bottle of Sèvres porcelain, and Étourdissant. But it was not until 1962 that he had a real success, when he produced Bal à Versailles. This was a brilliant oriental perfume with some 300 ingredients, mostly natural, and appeared in a series of polished crystal flasks designed by Pierre Dinand, with a label reproducing a painting by Fragonard. It was one of the most expensive perfumes ever marketed.

The company had more modest successes later from Jardanel (in 1973) and Sheherazade (1983), but in 1994 the firm was sold to an American-owned company, Parlux.

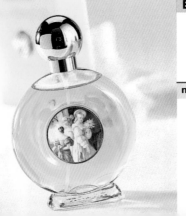

Bal à Versailles

LAUNCHED	*1962*
CREATOR	*Jean Desprez*
CATEGORY	*oriental amber spicy*
FLACON	*Pierre Dinand*

notes

TOP	*rose, jasmine, orange flower*
MIDDLE	*patchouli, sandalwood, vetiver*
LOWER	*musk, civet, amber*

PARFUMS CHRISTIAN DIOR

*One of the best-known names in perfumes that are innovative
and trendsetting*

PARENT COMPANY	*Louis Vuitton, Moët, Hennessy (LVMH)*
HEADQUARTERS	*Paris, France*
CURRENT PERFUMES	*Miss Dior, Diorissimo, Diorella, Dioressence, Poison, Dune, Tendre Poison, Dolce Vita, Eau Svelte, Hypnotic Poison*

Christian Dior established Parfums Dior with the launch of Miss Dior in 1947. He had always been attracted by fragrances. "I think of myself," he once said, "as a designer of perfumes as well as a designer of fashion," adding: "I became a perfumer so that one only has to open a bottle to imagine all my dresses, and so that each and every woman I dress leaves behind her an unforgettable aura."

He also once confessed that as a child he had never dreamed of becoming a dress-designer; his early memories of women were not of their dresses but of the perfumes they wore.

Dior, who came from Granville, in northwest France, studied to become a diplomat, but changed his mind in 1928 and opened an art gallery. In 1935 he

Miss Dior

LAUNCHED	*1947*
CREATOR	*Jean Carles (Roure) and Paul Vacher*
CATEGORY	*floral green chypre*
FLACON	*Guerry Colas; Marie-Christine de Sayn Wittgenstein*

notes

TOP	*gardenia, galbanum, clary sage, aldehydes*
MIDDLE	*jasmine, rose, neroli, narcissus, iris, carnation, lily of the valley*
LOWER	*patchouli, labdanum, oak moss, ambergris, sandalwood, vetiver, leather*

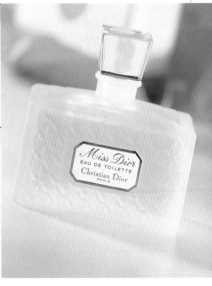

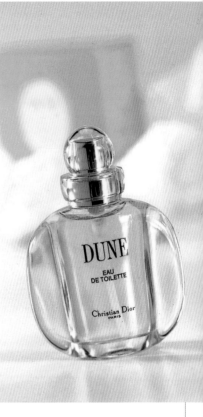

Dune

LAUNCHED *1991*

CREATOR *Jean-Louis Sieuzac (now Haarmann & Reimer)*

CATEGORY *floral oceanic*

FLACON *in-house, Véronique Monod and Marie-Christine de Sayn Wittgenstein*

notes

LINEAR *broom, wallflower, bergamot, mandarin, lily, peony, jasmine, rose, amber, lichen, musk, sandalwood, vanilla*

started to sell designs for hats, clothing, and accessories to the fashion houses and then worked briefly for the designer Robert Piguet, but with the outbreak of war he joined the army and, after the Franco-German armistice of 1940, became assistant to Lucien Lelong, whose collections he designed for several seasons.

In 1946 he opened his own house, presenting his first, sensational collection early in 1947. For years women had dreamed of wearing more feminine dresses. Now restrictions on materials had been removed and Dior was able to fulfill that dream. During the show the chief editor of *Harper's Bazaar* was heard to say to Dior, "It's quite a revolution, dear Christian. Your dresses have such a new look." The New Look at once established Dior as the king of fashion all over the world.

Christian Dior's first boutique in the USA opened in 1948 and in London in 1954. By that time his Paris headquarters alone was employing over 1,000 people. In the following year he took on the only design assistant he ever had, the young Yves St Laurent. Apart from demands for his couture, there were now many calls for costumes for famous film stars. But in October 1957 the great man died from a heart attack. He was only 52. Yves St Laurent took over as artistic director until called up for military service, when Marc Bohan succeeded him. The Parfums Dior company was bought up by what was to become LVMH in 1968.

Altogether Parfums Christian Dior has launched 18 fragrances, and the eminent perfumers who have been brought in to create Dior perfumes include Edmond Roudnitska (who has created six), Guy Robert, Jean-Louis Sieuzac, and Pierre Bourdon. The company manufactures its own fragrances, its main factory being at St Jean-de-Braye, France.

Dior perfumes are always innovative, designed to set new trends. Miss Dior, which first emerged in a beautiful amphora-shaped Baccarat flacon and subsequently in a bottle featuring the houndstooth design found in tweed material, introduced a new light-green note into a floral perfume. Dune, which won the 1993 FiFi award for best woman's fragrance, introduced the oceanic note which has been popular ever since and made it Dior's best-selling perfume. The originality of the award-winning Dolce Vita is shown in its complicated category: "floral fresh spicy and soft woody." The newly launched Hypnotic Poison, created by Annick Menardo of Firmenich, is being sold only as an *eau de toilette* (after an initial limited-edition *eau de parfum*) and comes into a new category, "amber, woody musky." The bottle for it was designed by the glassmakers Saint Gobain Desjonquères.

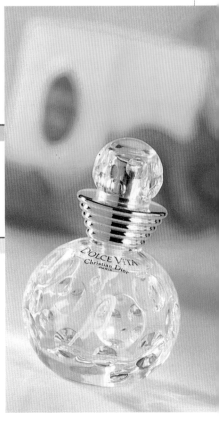

Dolce Vita

LAUNCHED	*1995*
CREATORS	*Pierre Bourdon with Maurice Roger*
CATEGORY	*fresh spicy floral and soft woody*
FLACON	*Serge Mansau*

notes

TOP	*lily, magnolia, rose*
MIDDLE	*apricot, cinnamon, peach*
LOWER	*sandalwood, heliotropin, vanilla*

DOLCE & GABBANA PARFUMS

Winner of the 1993 award for best female fragrance of the year

PARENT COMPANY	*EuroItalia*
HEADQUARTERS	*Milan, Italy*
CURRENT PERFUMES	*Dolce & Gabbana Parfum, By Dolce & Gabbana, D&G Feminine*

Domenico Dolce, from Sicily, and Stefano Gabbana, from Venice, are fashion designers who teamed up while working together in Milan. They have their own very individual approach to fashion, seeing it as unashamedly sexy and using sumptuous fabrics.

Having held their first women's show in 1986, they now design men's clothing as well, plus a wide range of extras, from ties to swimming suits, and have a strong Far East representation. In 1992 they formed Dolce & Gabbana Parfums and entered the perfume world with a high-quality fragrance called Dolce & Gabbana Parfum, which won the Accademia del Profumo's 1993 award for "best female fragrance of the year." This was followed in 1998 with a floral perfume called By Dolce & Gabbana, which seeks to stress the animal-like aspects of a woman's character; the effect is partly achieved by packaging with a leopardskin design.

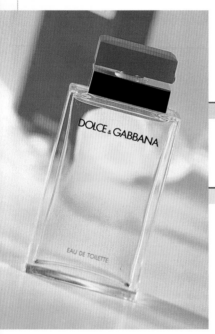

Dolce & Gabbana Parfum

LAUNCHED	*1992*
CREATORS	*IFF perfumers*
CATEGORY	*floral aldehyde*
FLACON	*Pierre Dinand*

notes

TOP	*petitgrain, tangerine, basil, ivy, freesia, aldehydes*
MIDDLE	*rose, orange flower, jasmine, carnation, lily of the valley, marigold, cilantro*
LOWER	*sandalwood, vanilla, tonka, musk*

PARFUMS D'ORSAY

The firm with a high reputation for exquisite perfumes and flacons

PARENT COMPANY	*Marignan*
HEADQUARTERS	*Paris, France*
CURRENT PERFUMES	*Etiquette Bleue, Arome 3, Tilleul, Intoxication d'Amour*

Etiquette Bleue

LAUNCHED	*1908 (relaunched 1993)*
CREATOR	*said to be from a formula by Count d'Orsay*
CATEGORY	*green aromatic*
FLACON	*Federico Rostrepo*

notes

TOP	*citrus, petitgrain, rosemary*
MIDDLE	*rosewood, orange flower*
LOWER	*sandalwood, balsam of Peru, oak moss*

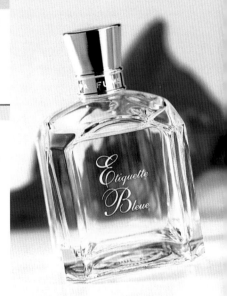

During the Napoleonic Wars, Count Alfred d'Orsay, a well-known dandy and romantic, was exiled to London because of his support for King Louis XVIII. There he had a passionate secret affair with a beautiful but married English aristocrat, Margaret, Countess of Blessington. His lover told him how she disliked the musky notes of fashionable perfumes, and he resolved to learn the perfumer's art and create a perfume to her taste. He called it L'Eau de Bouquet.

The formula was discovered some 50 years later in the d'Orsay family archives, when Parfums d'Orsay was established by a group of businessmen. Whether or not this link with the Count was a fiction, as some suppose, it is a fact that the new company, run by a remarkable woman, Madame Guerin, achieved a high reputation for exquisite perfumes and flacons.

The company fell into difficulties during the war, but was relaunched in Paris in 1993 by Alain Lagier. Its principal perfume, L'Eau de Bouquet, survives under the name Etiquette Bleue.

ESCADA

The company with a reputation for high-quality eaux de toilette

PARENT COMPANY	*independent*
HEADQUARTERS	*Munich, Germany*
CURRENT PERFUMES	*Escada, Escada Acte 2, Escada Sport, Sunny Frutti, Loving Bouquet*

Escada was the fashion label of the German designer Margaretha Ley and her husband Wolfgang Ley when they set up their fashion house in Munich in 1976. At that time they made knitwear to her designs, but they were soon producing a line of couture-quality sportswear which sold so well that it brought them into world prominence.

Margaretha died in 1992, but the company continued to expand its business and now owns over 170 stores, boutiques, and international showrooms, together with several other labels, which it has acquired as subsidiaries, including Cerruti 1881.

The foundation of Margaretha Ley's fragrance business was her Escada perfume, launched in 1990 when she opened her fragrance house, Escada Beauté Ltd. It was a richly feminine, very sensual fragrance marketed from the start at *parfum* and *eau de parfum* concentrations in elegant heart-shaped flacons of hand-blown crystal embellished

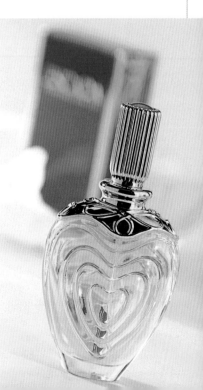

Escada

LAUNCHED	*1990*
CREATORS	*perfumers of Créations Aromatiques*
CATEGORY	*floral oriental*
FLACON	*Ken Kotyuk*

notes

TOP	*galbanum, bergamot, hyacinth, osmanthus, mandarin, peach, coconut*
MIDDLE	*orange flower, ylang-ylang, jasmine, carnation*
LOWER	*cedar, moss, vanilla*

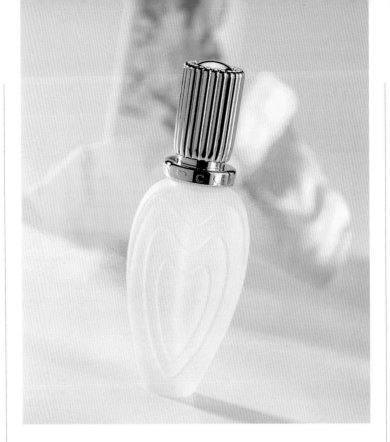

with swirls of gilded filigree. It has sold successfully ever since.

Escada Acte 2, described as a "multi-sensory" fragrance, with floral and ozonic notes, followed in 1995. But the company has also made a name for itself by producing a series of high-quality *eaux de toilette* to complement its annual spring/ summer fashion collection, each scent being withdrawn when the next is issued. These started with Chiffon Sorbet in 1993 and Summer in Provence in 1994. The 1998 version is Sunny Frutti, alcohol-free, which came out with a frosted green bottle and is advertised using the face of the company's own exclusive model, Pauline Poriskova. Scents from this series can sometimes be found in specialist perfume stores and are also available as a full set in a coffret of miniatures.

Sunny Frutti

LAUNCHED **1998**
CREATOR **n/a**
CATEGORY **fresh floral**
FLACON **Bernard Kotyuk**

notes

TOP **syringa, osmanthus, pear, nashi**
MIDDLE **apricot, freesia, lily of the valley, jasmine**
LOWER **cedar, moss, vanilla**

PARFUMS FENDI

The small store that became a major fashion house, now selling luxurious fragrances

PARENT COMPANY	*Florbath SA*
HEADQUARTERS	*Milan, Italy*
CURRENT PERFUMES	*Fendi, Asja, Fantasia, Theorema*

When Adele Fendi started up her business in Rome in 1925 she can have had little idea of the way it was going to develop. It was a small store selling fur and leather goods. As she grew older the running of it was taken over by her five daughters. It is now Fendi International, a major fashion house, with a perfume subsidiary until recently run by Sanofi and now acquired by the Italian company, Florbath SA.

The first Fendi perfume, called Fendi, came out in 1988 and in 1993 it launched Asja (pronounced "Asya"), a luxurious floral oriental named after "the Empress of Sensuality" and contained in a fiery-red, Japanese-style, glass flacon. In 1996 Fantasia, specifically tailored for the younger woman, was marketed in brightly colored bottles. The latest perfume from Parfums Fendi, launched at the end of 1998, is Theorema, designed to catch "the warmth of a Mediterranean sunset." It comes in a neat wedge-shaped bottle, reminiscent of the famous Fendi handbags, and the photography in the advertising, using the model Nadia Auermann as the "face," is by Karl Lagerfeld.

Theorema

LAUNCHED	*1998*
CREATOR	*Christine Nagel (Quest)*
CATEGORY	*floral oriental*
FLACON	*Catherine Krunas*

notes

TOP	*citrus, jasmine, eglantine*
MIDDLE	*osmanthus, cinnamon, pepper*
LOWER	*amber, macassar, sandalwood, cream*

FERREGAMO

From innovative and stylish shoes to quality perfumes

PARENT COMPANY	*Bvlgari*
HEADQUARTERS	*Geneva, Switzerland*
CURRENT PERFUME	*Salvatore Ferregamo pour Femme*

The position of this perfume house has changed considerably in recent years and the story provides a good example of what is happening in the perfume industry today. Salvatore Ferregamo entered the world of fashion as a maker of very innovative and stylish shoes and is credited with initiating the stiletto heel, the cork platform, and the invisible sandal. He became known as "the shoemaker to the stars." His interests spread to a variety of other products, including leather goods and silk accessories.

His company's first entry into the women's perfume market was with F de Ferregamo in 1971 and in 1994 it launched Ferregamo. In 1994 the Ferregamo family sold their fragrance company to Procter & Gamble. Two years later Ferregamo took over the distinguished perfume house of Ungaro (see page 179) from Chanel and subsequently joined up with Bvlgari (see page 55), leaving Procter & Gamble. The three are now jointly run by Bvlgari but retain their separate identities as perfume houses.

This is the background against which a new fragrance emerged from Ferregamo at the end of 1998 called Salvatore Ferregamo pour Femme, sold in a line up to full *parfum* concentration. Other fragrances are promised from the company.

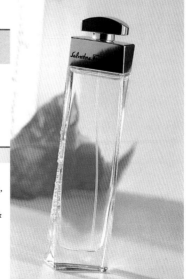

Salvatore Ferregamo pour Femme

LAUNCHED	*1998*
CREATOR	*Jacques Cavallier (Firmenich)*
CATEGORY	*floral*
FLACON	*Thierry de Bashmakoff*

notes

TOP	*anise, neroli, cassis*
MIDDLE	*iris, rose, peony, nutmeg, pepper*
LOWER	*raspberry, almond, musk*

FLORIS

Eight generations of perfumers to royalty and much of sophisticated London, the oldest perfume house in the world

PARENT COMPANY	*independent*
HEADQUARTERS	*London, England*
CURRENT PERFUMES	*Bouvardia, Edwardian Bouquet, Florissa, Gardenia, Lavender, Lily of the Valley, Seringa, Stephanotis, Zinnia*

Floris is the oldest major perfume house in the world. It was founded at a barber's shop in Jermyn Street, London, in 1730 by a young Spaniard, Juan Famenias Floris, shortly after he arrived from Minorca. Jermyn Street at that time was a narrow, cobbled thoroughfare, but its proximity to the Court of St James made it an ideal location for the young man, who was soon kept busy shaving the beards and powdering the wigs of illustrious visitors and residents.

But Floris had another vocation. He wanted to collect, mix, and sell some of the wonderful fragrances he could recollect from his youth in the Mediterranean. Very soon he was the perfumer to much of sophisticated London and in 1820 his son (for he married an English girl) received the company's first royal warrant.

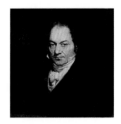

ABOVE: *Juan Famenias Floris.*

Floris still hold royal warrants to supply the British Queen and the Prince of Wales. The store is still there, too, with its elegant

Stephanotis

LAUNCHED	*eighteenth century*
CREATORS	*Floris perfumers*
CATEGORY	*single-note floral*
FLACON	*in-house*

notes

LINEAR	*orange blossom, carnation, jasmine, petitgrain, cilantro*

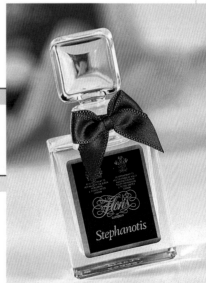

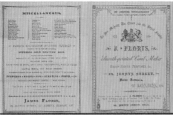

Gardenia

LAUNCHED **1996**
CREATORS **Floris perfumers**
CATEGORY **green floral**
FLACON **in-house**

notes

TOP **fresh green fruity**
MIDDLE **gardenia, lily,
cyclamen, tuberose,**
LOWER **jasmine**

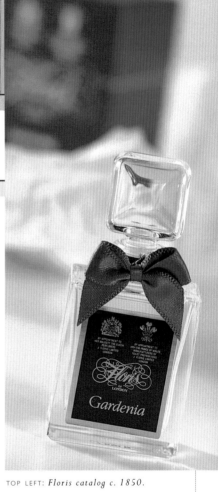

furnishings and mahogany display cases (survivors of the Great Exhibition of 1851), and members of the family, the eighth generation now, still sit in its paneled boardroom.

The business was passed down by marriage to the Bodenham family at the beginning of the twentieth century and has since expanded substantially. The company now has

TOP LEFT: *Floris catalog c. 1850.*

a large distribution center in Sussex, England, and runs a factory near Tiverton, in Devon, where all its own toiletries and fragrances are produced and where it also manufactures on contract for over 75 other companies. It exports worldwide and has its own stores in New York and in Kobe in central Japan.

The first fragrance sold by Juan Floris was Lavender. It is still being sold. But since that time dozens of other fragrances have been introduced and currently it is selling 15, including those for men, several others of which also date from the eighteenth century.

JEAN-PAUL GAULTIER

Creator of clothes, then fragrances, for the avant-garde

PARENT COMPANY	*Shiseido*
HEADQUARTERS	*Paris, France*
CURRENT PERFUMES	*Jean-Paul Gaultier, Summer Fragrance (limited edition)*

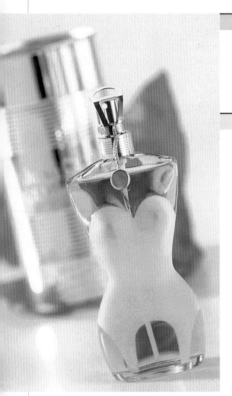

Jean-Paul Gaultier

1993
Jacques Cavallier
(Firmenich)
soft powdery floral
Jean-Paul Gaultier

notes

TOP *orange blossom, rose, tangerine, star anise*
MIDDLE *orchid, iris, ylang-ylang, ginger*
LOWER *vanilla, amber, musk*

At the age of 18 Jean-Paul Gaultier was working for Pierre Cardin, later for Jean Patou. A restless young man of the 1970s, he then went off to the Philippines, returning in 1976 to start designing clothes for the more avant-garde young. His enigmatic character has humor and curiosity, and his clothes belong to the Paris streets, with colors from the 1950s cinema.

It is against this background that one should evaluate his first perfume, Jean-Paul Gaultier (followed in 1997 by a complementary male fragrance). The perfume comes in a startling bottle showing a corseted female torso, somewhere between Madonna and Schiaparelli's Shocking, contained in a cylindrical tin can. In 1997 Gaultier also introduced Summer Fragrance, in a similar bottle but displaying a low-cut tattoo-motif dress over the corset. This fragrance is a limited edition.

ROMEO GIGLI

The minimalist and Byzantine who brings together the exotic and the classical

PARENT COMPANY	*Aeffe Spa*
HEADQUARTERS	*Milan, Italy*
CURRENT PERFUMES	*Romeo di Romeo Gigli, G. Gigli*

Romeo Gigli, born in Castelbolognese, Italy, approached fashion from an unusual background. His parents were antique book dealers and his education was in classical studies and architecture, enlivened by the travel that was a necessary part of the book trade, a love for which he inherited. He turned to fashion in New York, where he trained, subsequently returning to Italy, and was quickly successful. His first collection, in 1986, was highly acclaimed.

He has described himself as a minimalist and a Byzantine, which seems apt for a person who brings the exotic into a classical, artistic foundation. His fragrances include two for women, Romeo di Romeo Gigli and, for the young, G. Gigli. The former is one of the very first to be made using head space technology, in this case to enhance the freesia scent in the middle note. Colored pink, it comes in an intriguing bottle inspired by an eighteenth-century Venetian paperweight and won both a FiFi and an Italian Perfume Academy award.

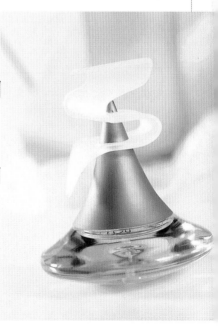

Romeo di Romeo Gigli

LAUNCHED	*1991*
CREATOR	*Sophie Labbé (IFF)*
CATEGORY	*floral*
FLACON	*Serge Mansau*

notes

TOP	*galbanum, basil, marigold, hesperides*
MIDDLE	*freesia, broom, orange blossom, rose, jasmine, lily of the valley, carnation*
LOWER	*frankincense, benzoin, orris, sandalwood*

GIORGIO BEVERLY HILLS

The firm that used new technology and created the "scent of the century"

PARENT COMPANY	*Procter & Gamble*
HEADQUARTERS	*California, USA*
CURRENT PERFUMES	*Giorgio, Wings, Red, Ocean Dream, Hugo for Women*

Giorgio Beverly Hills started off as a busy fashion boutique with white-and-yellow striped awnings established in Beverly Hills, California, in 1961 by Fred and Gale Hayman. They did well and eventually decided to launch a perfume, which came out in 1981 under the name Giorgio Beverly Hills, but is now called Giorgio, with white and yellow stripes on the packaging. This was a highly original fragrance, one of the first of the so-called linear fragrances devised in the 1980s, which replaced the classical pyramid structure with a long-lasting burst of notes. It was very strong, very heavy, very widely advertised (the first perfume to be promoted with scent strips inserted in magazines), and a huge success.

The Haymans were now in the world of big business and tempting offers came their way. In 1987 their perfume company was bought up, to the surprise of many, by the mass-market company Avon, founded in the USA in 1886, which sells from house to house through its "Avon ladies" and wished to obtain a stake in the top end of the market. Under Avon ownership another unusually strong perfume, Red, was launched in

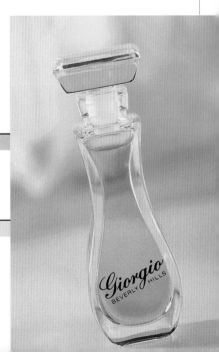

Giorgio

LAUNCHED *1981*
CREATOR *Florasynth perfumers*
CATEGORY *floral*
FLACON *n/a*

notes

LINEAR *rose, jasmine, gardenia, orange flower, sandalwood, patchouli, camomile*

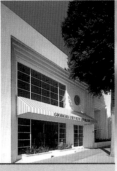

Wings

LAUNCHED *1993*

CREATOR *Jean-Claude Delville (IFF)*

CATEGORY *brilliant floriental*

FLACON *n/a*

notes

TOP *ginger lily, osmanthus, passion flower, gardenia, marigold, rose*

MIDDLE *orchid, jasmine, lilac, heliotrope, cyclamen*

LOWER *amber, musk, sandalwood, cedarwood*

ABOVE: *The original boutique, Rodeo Drive, Beverly Hills.*

1989, one of the first major perfumes to use the newly developed technique called headspace technology. It is said to contain 692 ingredients, falls into a new fragrance category called fleuriffe chypre, and was termed "the scent of the century."

While the house was still under Avon ownership, the highly successful Wings appeared in 1993, another very complicated IFF creation, with 621 ingredients, some produced by headspace technology. This introduced a vivid top note round ginger lily, the first major use of this plant in perfumery. The flacons for Wings were inspired by the great *Winged Victory* statue in the Louvre. But the ownership of Giorgio Beverly Hills was to change again. In 1994 it was acquired from Avon by Procter & Gamble, who remain the parent company.

In 1996 Giorgio Beverly Hills brought out a new women's fragrance, Ocean Dream, composed by melding ten accords of floral and oceanic notes into a scent designed to celebrate the lifestyle of southern California. In the

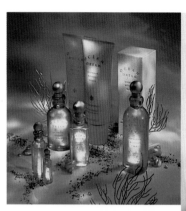

ABOVE: *Ocean Dream product range.*

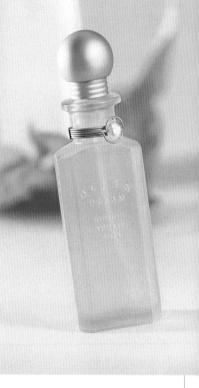

Ocean Dream

LAUNCHED **1996**

CREATOR **Alberto Morillas (Firmenich)**

CATEGORY **aquatic floral**

FLACON **n/a**

notes

LINEAR **water lily, water heliotrope, orange blossom, sandalwood, musk**

same year it started a line of limited-edition perfumes with Giorgio Aire, followed in 1998 by Holiday (in a neat, opaque coral-red bottle); no doubt there will be others. It also now runs other fragrance houses held by Procter & Gamble, notably the house of Laura Biagiotti, the distinguished Italian fashion designer, who had launched Laura Biagiotti in 1982, Roma in 1990, and Venezia in 1993 (of these only Roma is still being marketed). We may also soon hear more of the house of Herve Leger, the French designer, who recently formed a new perfume house in conjunction with Procter & Gamble to market further fine fragrances.

What, then, of the Haymans? They went their different commercial ways. Fred set up a successful new fragrance business under his own name in 1987, launching 272 for Women, In Love, and finally Touch, which included a perfume made as a compressed powder in a gold-plated compact. He sold this business to Parlux Fragrances in 1994. Gale founded a separate company, Gale Hayman Inc., which has launched other perfumes (see page 110).

PARFUMS GIVENCHY

The firm that designed the "perfume for a thousand women in one"

PARENT COMPANY	*Louis Vuitton, Moët, Hennessy (LVMH)*
HEADQUARTERS	*Paris, France*
CURRENT PERFUMES	*Organza, Organza Perfumed Summer Mist, L'Interdit, Givenchy III, Ysatis, Amarige, Fleur d'Interdit, Extravagance, Eau de Givenchy*

Parfums Givenchy was founded by Hubert de Givenchy in 1957, when he launched two famous perfumes simultaneously: Le de Givenchy (now called Le De) and L'Interdit. Givenchy was born in 1927 in Beauvais, in northern France, where his company now has a huge factory. He had started from small beginnings, with a family that would give him no encouragement to make a career in fashion as he wanted.

In 1945 he went to Paris to learn for himself by attending the Ecole des Beaux Arts as an unregistered student, and by working in a succession of famous designers' studios—Jacques Fath, Robert Piguet, Lucien Lelong, and Elsa Schiaperelli. Finally, he borrowed enough money to open his own fashion house with a staff of 15. In 1953 he presented his first collection, which was lavishly acclaimed. He launched his first ready-to-wear collection in 1956 and in 1958 he led the way with

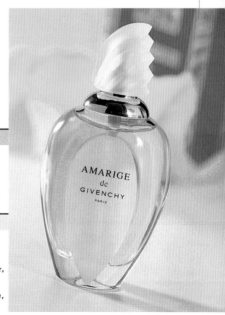

Amarige

LAUNCHED	*1991*
CREATOR	*Dominique Ropion*
CATEGORY	*floral woody*
FLACON	*Serge Mansau*

notes

TOP	*tangerine, violet, rosewood, neroli*
MIDDLE	*gardenia, mimosa, cassie, ylang-ylang*
LOWER	*ambergris, musk, vanilla, sandalwood, tonka*

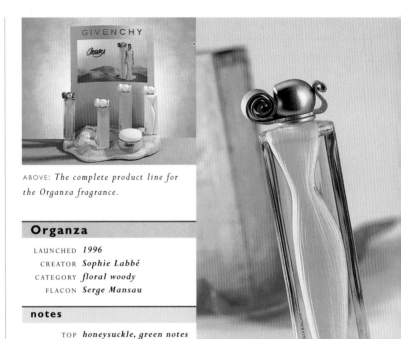

ABOVE: *The complete product line for the Organza fragrance.*

Organza

LAUNCHED **1996**
CREATOR **Sophie Labbé**
CATEGORY **floral woody**
FLACON **Serge Mansau**

notes

TOP **honeysuckle, green notes**
MIDDLE **gardenia, ylang-ylang, tuberose, peony**
LOWER **cedar, guaiac, sandalwood, vanilla, mace, nutmeg**

shorter skirts so that, for the first time since the 1920s, women could show their knees.

The year 1953 was a notable one for Hubert de Givenchy. Besides the success of his first collection, it also marked his first meeting with Cristobal Balenciaga, who had always been his idol and was from then on to become a lifelong friend. It marked, too, his meeting with Audrey Hepburn, who had seen his clothing and came to Paris to ask him to design costumes for her in the film *Sabrina*. She was to be one of his dearest friends and subsequently he designed many other film costumes for her (*Funny Face, Love in the Afternoon, Breakfast at Tiffany's*) as well as gowns for her personal wardrobe.

Givenchy was a compulsive designer and in his later years he has designed room interiors, wallpapers, carpets, furnishings, fabrics, china, bed linen, and tableware, including whole floors of some of the world's most prestigious hotels.

Givenchy's first two perfumes were immediately successful. L'Interdit is of course strongly associated with Audrey Hepburn, as a tribute to whom it was launched. Both are still available from specialist perfumers, but Le De is now made only as an *eau de toilette*.

Since then other notable Givenchy perfumes have followed. Ysatis, produced in 1984, should be mentioned in particular. It came at a time when French perfume houses were having to challenge foreign competition, and Parfums Givenchy had just been sold to another company, which was eventually to become the high-class luxury-goods concern Louis Vuitton, Moët, Hennessy (LVMH). The invented name was chosen because it sounded feminine and tied in with "Givenchy." The perfume, created by Dominique Ropion, was designed as "a perfume for a thousand women in one," with chypre, flowery, and oriental accords woven together. It started a new trend and is still one of the top bestsellers.

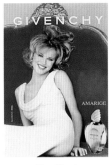

ABOVE: *Eva Herzigova, dressed in Givenchy haute couture.*

Amarige followed in 1991, a "white-flower" fragrance intended for a very feminine woman. Then came Organza, named after the material of which Hubert de Givenchy was so fond, and now the most popular of all Givenchy fragrances. Lastly Extravagance, the perfume for the Alexander McQueen era of Givenchy, intended to be sophisticated and aristocratic but not domineering, built on a basis of wisteria and launched on the face of the model Eva Herzigova.

Extravagance

LAUNCHED	*1998*
CREATOR	*Michel Girard*
CATEGORY	*green floral*
FLACON	*Serge Mansau*

notes

TOP	*green mandarin, tagetes, peppercorn, nettle*
MIDDLE	*jasmine, orange blossom, wisteria, wild strawberry, violet leaf*
LOWER	*sandalwood, cedarwood, amber, iris*

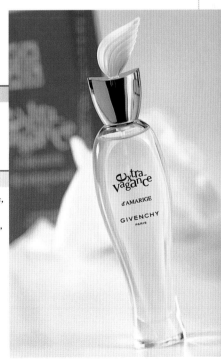

ANNICK GOUTAL

Creator of fragrances inspired by emotions, "or a very intense moment"

PARENT COMPANY	*Taittinger*
HEADQUARTERS	*Paris, France*
CURRENT PERFUMES	*Passion, Heure Exquise, Gardenia Passion, Rose Absolue, Grand Passion, plus others sold at* eau de toilette *strength*

This sophisticated perfumery was opened in a small boutique in Paris in 1980, shortly after Annick Goutal had created her first perfume, Fol Avril. She had trained to become a professional pianist, but realized at the age of 16 that perfumery was what she really wanted to do and gave up music to concentrate on it, marrying a perfumer from Grasse, France, in the process.

Her delicate, single-note compositions are made entirely from natural materials. "Each of my perfumes," she has said, "is inspired by an emotion, a time in my life, or a very intense moment." In 1986 her talent was recognized when she won an important *prix d'excellence* for European perfumes.

Altogether she has now launched 19 fragrances, which she sells from perfumeries, from prestige counters in major department stores like Harrods, Saks, and Nieman Marcus, and from her own stylish boutiques, with their ivory and gold decor, of which she has four in Paris alone.

Grand Amour

LAUNCHED	*1997*
CREATOR	*Annick Goutal*
CATEGORY	*floral amber musk*
FLACON	*Annick Goutal*

notes

LINEAR *rose, jasmine, mimosa, broom, heather, lily, honeysuckle, hyacinth, amber, vanilla, myrtle, musk*

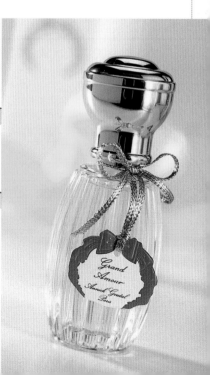

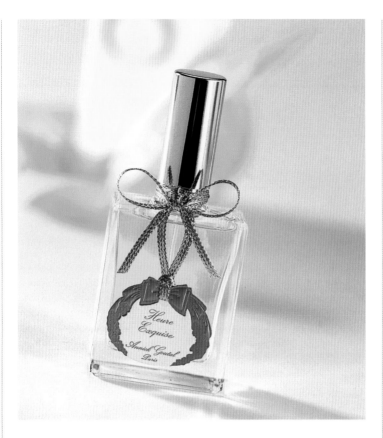

In the USA her success has been so considerable that the business is now run by a subsidiary company. She uses a signature flacon for most of her perfumes, spherical with a gilded glass butterfly on the stopper, which was designed after a scent bottle she found while exploring in an antiques store.

Heure Exquise

LAUNCHED *1980*
CREATOR *Annick Goutal*
CATEGORY *floral*
FLACON *Annick Goutal*

notes

LINEAR *based around rose, iris, and sandalwood*

Annick Goutal's principal perfumes for women are made at both *parfum* (*extrait*) and *eau de parfum* strength, as well as *eau de toilette*. They include Heure Exquise ("designed to give a gentle feeling like the transition of day into night"), Passion (warm and sensual, with tuberose, jasmine, and vanilla) and Grand Amour, her latest, which she has described as a scent of serene passion and which appears in a ruby-red version of her signature "butterfly" bottle.

PARFUMS GRÈS

*Creator of the award-winning perfume, Cabotine—a floral fragrance
with spicy overtones*

PARENT COMPANY	*Escada*
HEADQUARTERS	*Paris, France*
CURRENT PERFUMES	*Cabochard, Cabotine, Pastel de Cabotine, Folie Douce*

In the 1930s a sculptor and painter named Germaine Barton established a couture house in Paris which she merged in 1934 with another house called Maison Alix. At first she called the merged business Alix Barton Couture, but then, in 1942, she changed it to Alex Grès Couture. It was a long while before she introduced fragrance into her company, and during that period she came to be recognized as one of the most original designers of her time.

Then, in 1959, she took on Cabochard and launched it with a success that has continued ever since. Created by Bernard Chant (IFF), Cabochard is recognized as one of the most striking chypre perfumes to come on the market. It was first presented in a very simple bottle with a velvet bow, but the bow is now made of frosted glass. Unfortunately, as haute couture lost its clientele in the face of ready-to-wear, Madame Grès was obliged to prop up the profits of her couture business with those of the perfume.

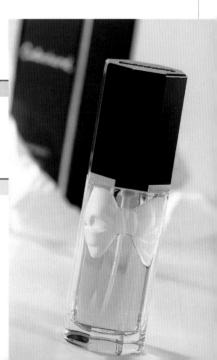

Cabochard

LAUNCHED	*1958*
CREATOR	*Bernard Chant (IFF)*
CATEGORY	*floral mossy chypre*
FLACON	*Jean Pérignon with Guighard Studio*

notes

TOP	*clary sage, galbanum, tarragon*
MIDDLE	*jasmine, rose, ylang-ylang*
LOWER	*oak moss, sandalwood, vetiver, patchouli*

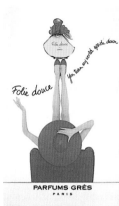

PARFUMS GRÈS
PARIS

Folie Douce

LAUNCHED *1998*
CREATORS *Sophie Labbé and Nathalie Lorson (IFF)*
CATEGORY *fruity floral*
FLACON *Serge Mansau*

notes

TOP *citrus, mimosa, blackcurrant*
MIDDLE *ylang-ylang, heliotrope, iris, lemon, bay*
LOWER *vanilla, cedar, musk, sandalwood*

ABOVE: *A daring advertisement for an unpredictable fragrance.*

Eventually there was inadequate capital left to carry on and she sold Parfums Grès to the British-American Tobacco Company in 1981.

She died aged 90 in 1993, but the perfume house has remained under various ownerships, ending up recently with Escada. In 1990 it issued the award-winning perfume Cabotine, a floral with spicy overtones created by Jean-Claude Delville (who was to create Wings a few years later) and presented in a flacon by Thierry Lecoule. Pastel de Cabotine followed, a floral fruity *eau de toilette* introduced in 1996. Finally Folie Douce appeared in 1998, with the *parfum* provided only in a gold purse spray decorated with roses.

PARFUMS GUCCI

The fragrance house with a line of distinguished perfumes behind it

PARENT COMPANY	*Wella*
HEADQUARTERS	*Paris, France*
CURRENT PERFUMES	*Eau de Gucci, Gucci No. 3, L'Arte de Gucci, Accenti, Envy*

The original business of Gucci was a leather factory, founded in Florence by Guccio Gucci in 1904 to produce saddles and harness. When hides were in short supply after World War I he started to make canvas luggage, and the business grew from there.

In 1993 the Gucci family gave up control and the fragrance wing of the company, Parfums Gucci, was bought by the German company Muelhens. Muelhens was then itself acquired by Wella. Their creative director—and significant influence behind all Gucci products—is now Tom Ford.

The fragrance house of Gucci has a line of distinguished perfumes behind it, including men's fragrances. It started with Gucci No. 1, created by a leading independent French perfumer, Guy Robert. Next, Parfums Gucci introduced Eau de Gucci, a floral perfume, in 1982. Gucci No. 3, launched in 1988 (there was no Gucci No. 2), is a floral aldehydic perfume.

L'Arte de Gucci, a floral oriental fragrance, appeared in 1992 and Accenti in 1995. Finally, in 1997, Gucci introduced Envy, which, having been heavily advertised and very well received, is on its way to being a substantial bestseller.

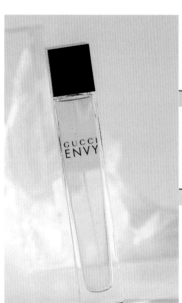

Envy

LAUNCHED	*1997*
CREATOR	*Maurice Roucel (Quest, now with Takasago)*
CATEGORY	*green floral*
FLACON	*Tom Ford*

notes

TOP	*hyacinth, magnolia, green notes*
MIDDLE	*lily of the valley, jasmine, violet*
LOWER	*iris, musk*

GUERLAIN

The perfumer who created fragrances for half the royal houses of Europe

PARENT COMPANY	*Louis Vuitton, Moët, Hennessy (LVMH)*
HEADQUARTERS	*Paris, France*
CURRENT PERFUMES	*Jicky, Aprés L'Ondée, L'Heure Bleue, Mitsouko, Shalimar, Liu, Vol de Nuit, Chant d'Arômes, Chamade, Parure, Nahema, Jardins de Bagatelle, Samsara, Un Air de Samsara, Champs-Élysées, Eau Impériale, Eau du Coq, Eau de Fleurs de Cedrat, Eau de Guerlain, Vega, Guerlinade*

Guerlain has so many top-class perfumes currently available that one can attempt to describe only a few of them in a book such as this. Indeed, since it started in 1828 the company has produced well over 300 fragrances. When Pierre-François-Pascal Guerlain opened his first little store in Paris he began by producing different personalized fragrances for each of his clients.

Paris was about to be reconstructed, with wide boulevardes being built. Soon he had premises in the newly fashionable Rue de la Paix and a factory at Colombes and, assisted by his two sons, Aimé and Gabriel, a growing reputation. He gained a royal warrant from the Queen of Belgium and, in 1853, after his Eau Impériale, with its Napoleonic bees decorating the

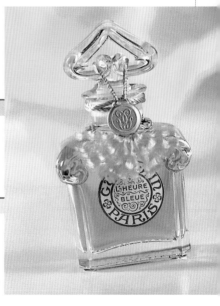

L'Heure Bleue

LAUNCHED	*1912*
CREATOR	*Jacques Guerlain*
CATEGORY	*semi-oriental powdery floral*
FLACON	*Raymond Guerlain*

notes

TOP	*bergamot, aniseed, neroli, tarragon*
MIDDLE	*carnation, jasmine, rose, neroli*
LOWER	*iris, vanilla, sandalwood, musk*

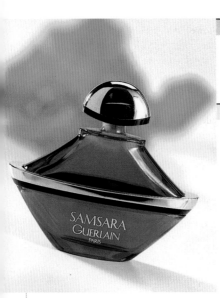

Samsara

LAUNCHED *1989*
CREATOR *Jean-Paul Guerlain*
CATEGORY *oriental woody floral*
FLACON *Robert Granai*

notes

TOP *jasmine*
MIDDLE *rose, narcissus, violet, orris, jasmine*
LOWER *sandalwood, tonka, iris, vanilla*

bottle, had delighted the Empress Eugénie, he was appointed His Majesty's Official Perfumer. That fragrance is still being sold.

He went on to provide perfumes for half the royal houses in Europe. "Make good products," Pierre-François-Pascal Guerlain impressed on his workers. "Never compromise on quality. For the rest, stick to simple ideas and apply them scrupulously." That guiding principle is still adhered to in the House of Guerlain.

Aimé inherited his father's creative bent and only five years after the old man's death, in 1889, he created Jicky, a perfume so different from what had come before, so trend-setting, so innovative, that it is known as the first modern perfume and regarded as one of the greatest of all perfume classics. The notes of Jicky, classified as a semi-oriental fougère fragrance, are quite uncomplicated by today's standards, but it introduced the major division into separate tiers of notes and for the first time it made proper use of materials that had been produced synthetically.

It was called Jicky because that was the name of an early girlfriend of Aimé's and was, too, Jacques Guerlain's nickname. The flacon, designed by another Guerlain and made by Baccarat, resembled an old chemist's bottle, with the stopper made to look like a champagne cork to symbolize the perfume's sparkle and happiness. Oddly enough, nobody ever decided whether it should be for men or for women, for there was little distinction in those times, and Jicky has remained a unisex (but perhaps mainly female) scent ever since.

It was Gabriel's sons who led the company next, with Jacques inheriting the wonderfully instinctive Guerlain nose for creating fragrances. A larger factory was developed and built and, in 1906, Jacques Guerlain created another timeless perfume, Aprés l'Ondée, followed swiftly by the famous, innovative floral-oriental L'Heure Bleue, a gift to his wife and a commercial challenge to Coty's L'Origan.

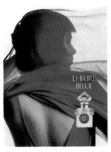

ABOVE: *Striking color of the blue hour.*

There followed that period between the wars when, for the rich, all life seemed to be a celebration. It produced Mitsouko, reflecting Puccini and Japan, Shalimar for the Orient, Liu, inspired by a character in *Turandot*, and Vol de Nuit, a salute both to aviation and to the cinema. Guerlain's trade was expanding all the time and new subsidiaries were being opened in other countries.

But wartime bombing smashed Guerlain factories and postwar recovery was unavoidably slow. In 1955 Jacques Guerlain created his last fragrance in conjunction with his grandson Jean-Paul, heir to the Guerlain gift—the Guerlain nose. Chamade, associated with beating drums, hearts, and surrender, followed in 1969; a fresh, tender scent, L'Eau de Guerlain, in 1974; a timeless chypre, Parure, in 1975; and Nahema, dedicated to the rose, in 1979. More recently have come Jardins de Bagatelle, a floral bouquet inspired by Tuscan music; then the floral oriental Samsara; the fresher, lighter, more zesty Un Air de Samsara; and, in 1996, the last so far of Jean-Paul Guerlain's great range of perfumes, Champs Élysées, which has innovative floral notes based on mimosa, mimosa leaves, and buddleia.

Champs-Élysées comes in a bottle by Robert Granai, who has designed all the Guerlain flacons since 1959, but in 1997 Guerlain introduced a new version of Vega, which they had first issued in 1936, in a limited-edition flacon made by Baccarat, and in 1998 a limited-edition perfume, Guerlinade, to mark the 200th anniversary of their founder's birth.

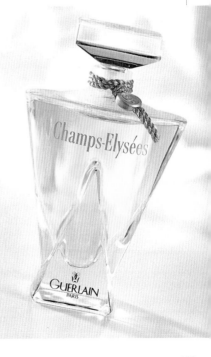

Champs-Élysées

LAUNCHED *1996*
CREATOR *Jean-Paul Guerlain*
CATEGORY *floral sparkling*
FLACON *Robert Granai*

notes

TOP *rose, blackcurrant, almond, mimosa leaves*
MIDDLE *mimosa, buddleia*
LOWER *hibiscus, almond wood*

GALE HAYMAN INC.

A famous name in the perfume world

PARENT COMPANY	*La Parfumerie Inc., New York*
HEADQUARTERS	*New York, USA*
CURRENT PERFUMES	*Delicious, Delicious Feelings, Sunset Boulevard*

Gale Hayman used to run a fashion boutique in Beverly Hills with her husband Fred, which they founded in 1961. Twenty years later they launched their first perfume, called Giorgio Beverly Hills, which did so well that their perfume company was bought, name and all, by Avon and has had an exciting history ever since (see page 96).

Fortune made, they might have been expected to retire, but instead each stepped back again, seperately, into the perfume business. Gale Hayman, forming Gale Hayman Inc., launched another successful perfume, Delicious, in 1994, and followed it up with Delicious Feelings in 1995. Delicious, a floral oriental perfume, comes in an interesting bottle showing a stylized rock surmounted by a snow leopard; the product was nominated for a FiFi award. Delicious Feelings, a lighter, floral scent made up to *eau de toilette* concentration, uses the same bottle.

A new floral *eau de toilette* fragrance, Sunset Boulevard, was launched by the company in 1998.

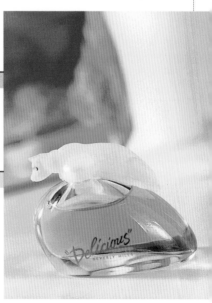

Delicious

LAUNCHED	*1994*
CREATOR	*René Morganthaler (Givaudan-Roure)*
CATEGORY	*floral oriental*
FLACON	*Gale Hayman*

notes

TOP	*narcissus, boronia, mimosa, mandarin, neroli, cassis*
MIDDLE	*rose, jasmine, tuberose, muguet, ylang-ylang, angelica*
LOWER	*sandalwood, patchouli, orris, musk*

HERMÈS PARFUMS

The company that values the quality of its raw materials for fragrances of nobility and glamour

PARENT COMPANY	*independent*
HEADQUARTERS	*Paris, France*
CURRENT PERFUMES	*Calèche, Amazone, Parfum d'Hermès, 24 Faubourg, Hermès Eau d'Orange (unisex), Eau d'Hermès (unisex)*

Hermès has been in business since 1837, when a saddle-maker, Thierry Hermès, moved to Paris and built up a steady trade making and selling saddles and harness. In 1879 his son moved into the famous address at 24, Faubourg St Honoré where Hermès remain. From a base of making leatherware products the company expanded, particularly under Émile Hermès early this century, to luggage, watches, clothing, and much else, altogether the products of 14 crafts and always of immaculate quality. The first of its silk scarves was introduced in 1937.

Expansion has been especially marked since 1978, when Jean-Louis Dumas succeeded his father at its head, and the business is now a very large one indeed, with over 250 stores worldwide, but it remains under family ownership and hence retains a human scale.

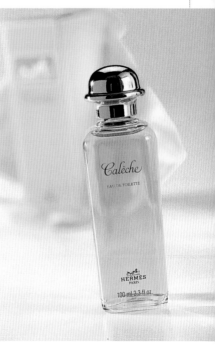

Calèche

LAUNCHED	*1961*
CREATOR	*Guy Robert*
CATEGORY	*floral woody chypre*
FLACON	*in-house*

notes

TOP	*bergamot, mandarin, orange blossom, aldehydes*
MIDDLE	*jasmine, lily of the valley, rose, gardenia, iris, ylang-ylang*
LOWER	*oak moss, sandalwood, cedar, vetiver*

24, Faubourg

LAUNCHED *1995*
CREATOR *Maurice Roucel (Quest)*
with Bernard Bourjois
CATEGORY *floral woody amber*
FLACON *Serge Mansau*

notes

LINEAR *orange blossom,*
jasmine, tiara flower,
ylang-ylang, iris,
patchouli, vanilla,
ambergris, sandalwood

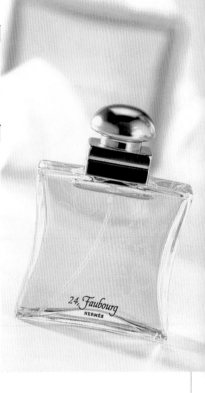

The company's fragrance house was opened in 1950, but its first big perfume did not emerge for 10 years. It functions from a factory complex at Veaudreuil, near Rouen, where it prepares its own fragrances under its own in-house perfumer, Bernard Bourjois.

Quality is an outstanding feature of all items from Hermès, who believe that "A fragrance's nobility, richness, and glamour are based on the quality of the natural, precious raw materials used to make it." There is no stinting with a Hermès product.

The first few of the Hermès perfumes were house scents, sold only from Hermès stores, but Eau d'Hermès, launched in 1951, was a refined unisex fragrance created by the great Edmond Roudnitska and is still available. Then in 1960 came Calèche, which was created by Guy Robert just after he had devised Madame Rochas. The bottle showed a stylish carriage on the label, a *grand duc*, in fact, rather than the *calèche*, which is the Hermès symbol. This scent was to become an enduring classic.

CAROLINA HERRERA PERFUMES

The house of fashion and fragrance, cosmetics and accessories

PARENT COMPANY	*Antonio Puig*
HEADQUARTERS	*New York, USA*
CURRENT PERFUMES	*Carolina Herrera, Flore, 212, Carolina Herrera*

The fragrance house of Carolina Herrera belongs to Puig. Antonio Puig (pronounced "pooch") founded his company in Barcelona in 1914 as an agency importing French fragrances into Spain. In the 1920s he began to make his own brands and developed the first lipstick to be produced in Spain, but his big success was a toilet water, Agua Lavanda, launched in 1940. Antonio Puig died in 1979 at the age of 90, leaving sons and grandchildren to run the business, which is now a multimillion-dollar one in the field of fragrances, soaps, toiletries, and baby products. Its huge manufacturing plant is the largest in Spain.

Fragrances exported under the Puig label are for men, although some perfumes for women, such as Estivalia and Tess, are made for the home market. Outside Spain the company's perfumes for women are found under the labels of Paris-based Paco Rabanne, which was set up in the 1970s, and New York-based Carolina Herrera, whose fragrance business it established with her in 1988. In 1998 the company also acquired Nina Ricci.

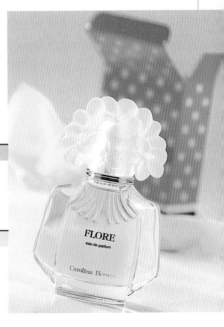

Flore

LAUNCHED	*1995*
CREATOR	*Dr Rosendo Mateu*
CATEGORY	*fresh floral aqueous*
FLACON	*André Ricard*

notes

TOP	*floral notes*
MIDDLE	*lily of the valley, iris, jasmine*
LOWER	*iris, musk, sandalwood, woody notes*

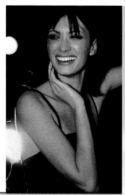

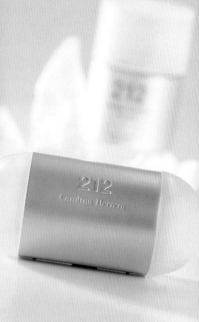

212, Carolina Herrera

LAUNCHED *1998*
CREATOR *Ann Gottlieb (IFF)*
CATEGORY *light floral*
FLACON *Fabien Baron*

notes

TOP *gardenia, cactus flower, bergamot*
MIDDLE *rose, camellia, lily, lace flower*
LOWER *satinwood, sandalwood, musk*

TOP LEFT: *212, "the hot new code in fragrance."*

Carolina Herrera is from Venezuela, where she lives in a sixteenth-century mansion. She comes from a rich, land-owning family and grew up in a world where women wore only couture clothing. Interested in fashion, she was encouraged to design it and her high standards and striking sense of style brought her great success. She now heads an international fashion design business based in New York, selling not only clothing but fragrances, cosmetics, and accessories as well. Perfume was introduced in 1988, when she linked up with Antonio Puig to launch a signature fragrance, Carolina Herrera, a single-note perfume based on a favorite blending of jasmine, tuberose, and nard, which she used to make for herself as a girl. Flore followed, a new category of floral fragrance composed using head space technology and built on iris, jasmine, and a green note, with a bottle depicting a floral bouquet in a vase. This was followed in 1997 by a lighter counterpart called Aqua Flore, and more recently 212, Carolina Herrera was launched, a floral *eau de toilette* made to provide "an ethereal, radiant effect." It comes in an unusual flacon which turns out to be two atomizers in one, the first for home and the second for the purse.

HOUBIGANT

The great French perfume house that created Quelques Fleurs—and a new fashion

PARENT COMPANY	*part owned by Renaissance Cosmetics*
HEADQUARTERS	*Paris, France, and Massachusetts, USA*
CURRENT PERFUMES	*Quelques Fleurs, Demi-Jour, Chantilly, Raffinée, Lutèce, French Vanilla, White Chantilly and others*

Houbigant is now no more than a shadow of its former self, for most of it has been torn away from the mother company and sold. But what is left can still claim to be the oldest of all the great French perfume houses. There was a time when this famous company, established in 1775 by Jean-François Houbigant when he was only 23, led the world with its toilet waters, powders, and scented gloves.

It is said that, before fleeing from Paris, Queen Marie Antoinette had hurried to Houbigant to get her perfume bottles refilled. Eau de Mousseline and Eau de Millefleurs had perfumed her courtiers. The company survived the turmoil of the French Revolution and, in 1807, passed on to Jean-François's son and then to Chardin, his partner, who was appointed as the personal perfumer to Napoleon.

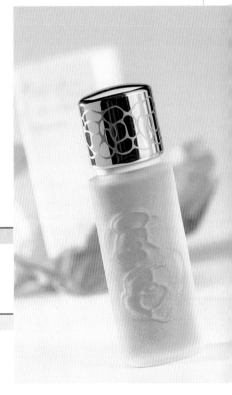

Quelques Fleurs

LAUNCHED	*1912, relaunched 1988*
CREATOR	*Robert Bienaimé*
CATEGORY	*floral*
FLACON	*n/a*

notes

TOP	*bergamot*
MIDDLE	*lilac, rose, jasmine, orchid*
LOWER	*amber, sandalwood*

Raffinée

LAUNCHED *1982*
CREATOR *Houbigant perfumers*
CATEGORY *floral oriental*
FLACON *Alain de Mourgues*

notes

TOP *jasmine, rose,
carnation, citrus*
MIDDLE *hyacinth, mimosa, orris,
tonka*
LOWER *frankincense, cypress,
sandalwood*

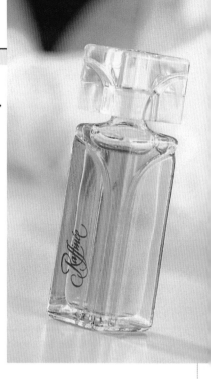

Josephine patronized the Houbigant boutique, and when Napoleon lay dying two of Houbigant's perfumed pastilles were burning in his bedroom. Queen Victoria, Napoleon III, and, in 1890, the Tsar of Russia all appointed Houbigant as their royal perfumer.

In 1880 the company was acquired by Paul Parquet, one of the first to use synthetics in his creations and the creator of the first fougère fragrance, Fougère Royale. At the turn of the century another eminent perfumer joined Houbigant, Robert Bienaimé, creator of the classic Quelques Fleurs, which was to prove to be the company's greatest success. One of the most notable perfumes ever made and often regarded as the first true multifloral scent, Quelques Fleurs started up a fashion for this type of fragrance.

New perfumes emerged from Houbigant regularly throughout the 1920s and 1930s, and Chantilly was launched in Paris during the war itself, but the company never got over the difficulties brought about by World War II and the subsequent days of economic hardship. A major effort was put into the business with new finance during the 1980s, when Ciao, Raffinée, Les Fleurs, Lutèce, and Demi-Jour were all launched, but it was not sufficient and more drastic steps had to be taken. Accordingly, in 1994 the rights to produce 12 of the main Houbigant scents, including the award-winning Raffinée, Chantilly, and Lutèce, were purchased by an American company, Renaissance Cosmetics, leaving Houbigant to concentrate on Quelques Fleurs (relaunched in 1988 in a bottle decorated with stylized flower petals) and Demi-Jour.

ICEBERG

Creator of cool fragrances with versions for both men and women

PARENT COMPANY	*Eurocosmesi*
HEADQUARTERS	*Milan, Italy*
CURRENT PERFUMES	*Iceberg Twice, Iceberg Twice Ice, Iceberg Universe*

Rather strangely for its name, Iceberg is a perfume house set up by an Italian fashion company, Gilmar, which Silvio Gerani and his designer wife Giulana established in 1960. It has its own boutiques all over the world, with particular interest in the Far East, and has launched several fragrances, but these days it is controlled by the big Italian fragrance company Eurocosmesi, itself a part of the Guaber Group.

Iceberg began selling perfumes in 1988 with Iceberg Parfum. This fragrance is no longer generally available on the market, but in 1995 the company came up with Iceberg Twice, following that in 1996 with Iceberg Twice Ice and in 1997 with Iceberg Universe, which is dedicated to the young. All these fragrances are made with men's versions to complement those for women. Twice Ice can be worn day or night, summer or winter. Designed to be fresh and bubbly, it starts with a cold note from litchis and contains an unusual dash of coffee in the dry-out to give it a warm ending.

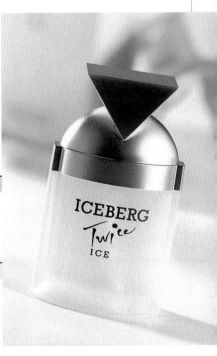

Iceberg Twice Ice

LAUNCHED	*1996*
CREATORS	*Quest Perfumers*
CATEGORY	*floral fruity*
FLACON	*Pierre Dinand*

notes

TOP	*litchi, rhubarb, bergamot*
MIDDLE	*jasmine, rose, lotus*
LOWER	*coffee, musk, amber, vanilla*

PERFUMES ISABELL

The former florist whose fragrances say it with flowers

PARENT COMPANY	*independent*
HEADQUARTERS	*New York, USA*
CURRENT PERFUMES	*Attar, Calla, Ceylon, Mandarin, Savanna*

This is a small New York perfume business which has recently come into prominence. Robert Isabell is well known in the international jet set as the man from New York who designs and stages lavish parties for the rich and famous—Alexandra Miller's wedding to Prince Alexander von Furstenburg in New York, Madonna's birthday party at a Miami Beach hotel.

Apprenticed to a florist in Minnesota, he moved to New York in 1978, where he worked for Renny, the town's leading florist, and Bergdorf Goodman. In setting up parties his special *métier* is the lavish use of flowers, with which he is infatuated, studying them all over the world.

After a period spent learning aspects of perfumery at the Givaudan-Roure laboratories in Zürich, he set up Perfumes Isabell in New York to market a range of five single-flower floral fragrances (there are now more) created through headspace technology. These are now also being sold at Harvey Nichols in London. The fragrances, which have the brilliant clarity of this "living flower" system, come in plain, tall cylindrical flasks.

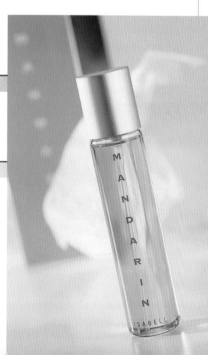

Mandarin

LAUNCHED	*1997*
CREATOR	*Robert Isabell*
CATEGORY	*floral citrus*
FLACON	*Takaai Matusmoto*

notes

TOP	*mandarin, lemon, lime, fresh green notes*
MIDDLE	*pomelo, jasmine, birch leaf, juniper berry, orange flower, cinnamon leaf*
LOWER	*musk, sandalwood, gur jum balsam*

PARFUMS JOOP!

Creator of the tempting fragrance redolent of the Garden of Eden

PARENT COMPANY	*Lancaster/Coty*
HEADQUARTERS	*Paris, France*
CURRENT PERFUMES	*Joop! Femme, All About Eve*

Parfums Joop! (always with the exclamation mark) began as the fragrance division of the international fashion empire built up by the Potsdam-born, Hamburg-based fashion designer Wolfgang Joop and his wife from 1981. As well as fashion and jeans, their business now also covers leather, knitwear, and many other accessories. For a time Wolfgang Joop was editor of the German fashion magazine *Neue Mode*. Parfums Joop! now belongs to the Lancaster group, which is a part of Coty.

Joop!'s first fragrance was Joop! Femme, an oriental perfume created by Takasago perfumers and introduced in 1987. For women Berlin was then launched in 1991 and Nightflight in 1992. But the company's best-selling fragrance is now All About Eve, which was launched in 1996. You can hardly think of Eve without an apple and this scent, designed to reflect her seduction in the Garden of Eden, is made up to full *parfum* concentration. The fragrance has a prominent apple note among the garden scents and appears in an apple-shaped flacon.

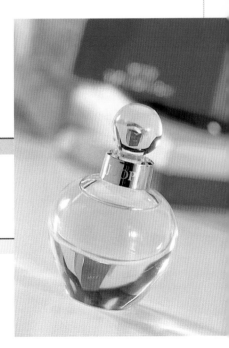

All About Eve

LAUNCHED	*1996*
CREATOR	*Perfumers of Créations Aromatique*
CATEGORY	*fruity floral*
FLACON	*Peter Schmidt*

notes

TOP	*apple, floral notes*
MIDDLE	*jasmine, cinnamon*
LOWER	*vetiver, vanilla*

JOSEPH

The nose for fashion that brought us the successful Parfum du Jour

PARENT COMPANY	*independent*
HEADQUARTERS	*London, England*
CURRENT PERFUME	*Parfum de Jour*

Joseph Ettedgui's highly respected position as a leading member of the London fashion world comes from a career that began in the 1960s, when he moved from Casablanca, his 1938 birthplace, opened an *avant-garde* hairdressing salon in London's King's Road and, late in the 1970s, converted to selling fashionable knitwear.

By the 1980s his clothes and stores were style leaders, his Joseph Tricot knitwear label being known all round the world, and he was being called "the man who made the decade." By 1994 he had been voted knitwear designer of the year four times. He now runs 17 Joseph fashion stores in London, New York, Paris, and elsewhere. He has a legendary nose for the next fashion trend.

In 1985 Joseph launched Parfum du Jour, in a small black bottle sold only from his own stores. This was relaunched in 1997 very successfully, for wider sales, with the same formula, which has over 100 ingredients, as an *eau de parfum*. The innovative new bottle has a photographic image of a woman's nose and lips screen-printed on the clear glass surface.

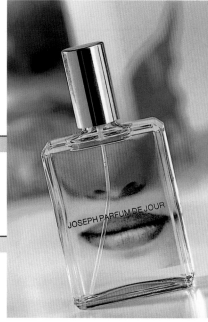

Parfum de Jour

LAUNCHED	*1985, relaunched 1997*
CREATOR	*perfumers of Penhaligon's*
CATEGORY	*floral*
FLACON	*Teresa Roviras*

notes

TOP	*mandarin, cassis*
MIDDLE	*jasmine, rose, hyacinth, muguet, ylang-ylang*
LOWER	*sandalwood, amber*

DONNA KARAN BEAUTY

One of America's leading perfume houses, the award-winning creator of Chaos

PARENT COMPANY	*Estée Lauder*
HEADQUARTERS	*New York, USA*
CURRENT PERFUMES	*Donna Karan New York, Chaos, Watermint (brand)*

Donna Karan New York

LAUNCHED	*1992*
CREATORS	*IFF perfumers*
CATEGORY	*floral amber spicy*
FLACON	*Stephen Weiss*

notes

LINEAR	*lily, ylang-ylang, rose, jasmine, heliotrope, apricot, cassia, patchouli, sandalwood, frankincense, amber, vanilla, musk*

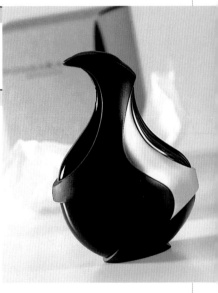

Donna Karan set up her fashion design company in New York in 1985 with her husband Stephen Weiss, but it was not until 1991 that the pair founded the Donna Karan Beauty Company and launched their first perfume, called Donna Karan New York. Stephen, a painter and sculptor, designed the bottle himself—an innovative black and gold abstract shape, sensual, modern, strong yet feminine, with the curves of a woman's body.

The perfume was issued in a line up to full-strength *parfum* concentration, with the usual variation of the bottle-shapes for the different items in the line. In 1993 it took the top FiFi award for Best Woman's Fragrance, together with the Best National Advertising Print Company award at the same ceremony, guaranteeing its all-round instant success.

Now established as one of America's leading perfume houses, Donna Karan has subsequently launched a new women's fragrance, Chaos, with notes of herbs and incense, first issued in 1997, and a new brand of fragrance, called Watermint, is also being presented.

PARFUMS KENZO

Fragrances of East and West—and a walk on the wild side

PARENT COMPANY	*Louis Vuitton, Moët, Hennessy (LVMH)*
HEADQUARTERS	*Paris, France*
CURRENT PERFUMES	*Kenzo, Parfum d'Été, Kashâya, L'Eau par Kenzo, Kenzo Jungle*

Back in the 1970s the Japanese designer Kenzo started a fashion business in Paris, France, and in 1988 he began to market a range of high-quality perfumes through his fragrance division, Parfums Kenzo. First was Kenzo itself, a bouquet of flowers and fruit created for him by Françoise Caron with a bottle shaped to resemble a beach pebble. Then came Parfum d'Été, a brilliant evocation of a summer's day with a flacon shaped like a leaf.

The division was subsequently acquired by the luxury group LVMH, which also owns the houses of Dior, Guerlain, and Givenchy. In 1994 it produced Kashâya, an oriental perfume in a bottle depicting leaves entwined as a symbol of love, and in 1996 came L'Eau par Kenzo, a floral, watery fragrance. Lastly, celebrating the Chinese Year of the Tiger in 1998, Kenzo Jungle was launched, an oriental described as a wild yet mild harmony.

Parfum d'Été

LAUNCHED	*1993*
CREATOR	*Christian Mathieu (IFF)*
CATEGORY	*floral*
FLACON	*Serge Mansau*

notes

TOP	*green and floral*
MIDDLE	*rose, jasmine, peony, narcissus, freesia, hyacinth*
LOWER	*musk, amber, sandalwood, oak moss*

CALVIN KLEIN

A diverse range of modern, innovative fragrances for today's woman

PARENT COMPANY	*Unilever*
HEADQUARTERS	*New York, USA*
CURRENT PERFUMES	*Obsession, Eternity, Escape, CK One (unisex), CK Be (unisex), Contradiction*

Calvin Klein was a well-established designer of 15 years' standing before his New York-based company launched its first fragrance, Obsession, in 1985. He had started his business with a childhood friend, Barry Schwartz, in 1968, initially designing coats and men's suits, then expanding to sportswear, jeans, hosiery, and accessories. By the mid-1980s producing a fragrance must have seemed a logical step forward. Calvin Klein Cosmetics Company was formed in 1985 with the launch of Obsession.

Obsession had a huge impact. It was totally modern, strong in composition, heavily advertised and overtly sexual in tone. "I wanted to evoke the sensuality and sexual ardor of an impassioned woman," said Klein. It was presented in an attractive, sensual flacon by Pierre Dinand, the foremost scent-bottle designer of

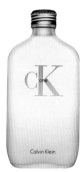

ABOVE: *CK One, a fragrance innovation.*

Obsession

LAUNCHED	*1985*
CREATOR	*Jen Guichard (Roure)*
CATEGORY	*floral oriental*
FLACON	*Pierre Dinand*

notes

TOP	*mandarin, bergamot, vanilla*
MIDDLE	*jasmine, orange blossom, sandalwood, vetiver, and spicy notes*
LOWER	*amber, oak moss, frankincense, musk*

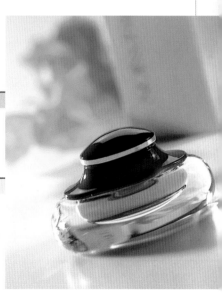

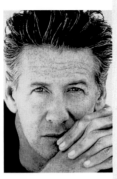

ABOVE: *Calvin Klein.*

Contradiction

LAUNCHED	*1997*
CREATOR	*Givaudan Roure perfumers*
CATEGORY	*oriental*
FLACON	*Fabien Baron*

notes

TOP	*eucalyptus, pepper flower, syringa, orchid*
MIDDLE	*muguet, jasmine, rose, peony*
LOWER	*tonka, sandalwood, satinwood*

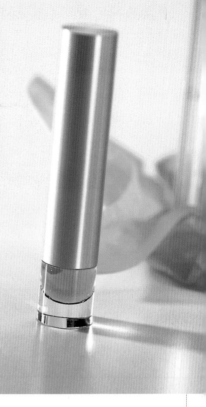

the present day, and it won a top American Fragrance Foundation (FiFi) award for "the most successful woman's fragrance." It was soon selling widely all round the world.

Over the next few years Calvin Klein produced two more successful fragrances, Eternity, a romantic bouquet celebrating his own wedding, and Escape, "for the romantic woman who wants to make every moment count," and complemented all three with equivalent men's fragrances.

Then, in 1994, came an innovation in the world of fine fragrance, CK One, a unisex *eau de toilette* with a green-tea accord in a plain, recyclable glass container shaped like a rum bottle. The launch of this scent was followed rapidly by CK Be, a more floral and musky unisex *eau de toilette* in a black but similarly shaped bottle. Finally, Calvin Klein has stepped back into the past with a complex, more traditionally feminine, oriental perfume called Contradiction, presented in an elegant cylindrical flacon; this is made up to full *parfum* concentration and was launched on the face of the model Christy Turlington. Every one of Calvin Klein's fragrances has won a FiFi award. All have been innovative, controversial successes.

PARFUMS KARL LAGERFELD

The perfumer who put heavenly bodies into the world of fragrance

PARENT COMPANY	*Elizabeth Arden / Unilever*
HEADQUARTERS	*New York, USA*
CURRENT PERFUMES	*Sun, Moon, Stars*

Karl Lagerfeld, who was born in 1939 of Swedish-German parents, has had a wide career at the very top of the fashion industry (and also in photography) and this is reflected in his associations in the perfume world, where his name recurs in different contexts. At various times he has worked for Balmain, Jean Patou, the House of Chloé, and Chanel, besides producing many collections in his own name.

While head designer for Chloé (see page 69) he persuaded them in 1975 to launch their own perfume, Chloé, and a little later established his own perfume house, Parfums Karl Lagerfeld (now run by Elizabeth Arden), launching an oriental perfume, KL (created by Roger Pellegrino of Firmenich), in 1982. His greatest perfume success has been Sun, Moon, Stars, created by a distinguished IFF perfumer, which comes in a blue spherical bottle patterned with a moon and stars and surmounted by a gold-colored, sun-shaped cap.

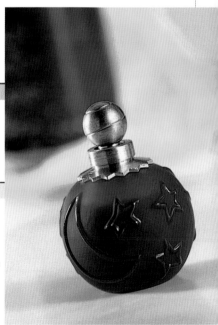

Sun, Moon, Stars

LAUNCHED	*1994*
CREATOR	*Sophia Grosjman (IFF)*
CATEGORY	*fruity floral oriental*
FLACON	*Karl Lagerfeld and Susan Wacker*

notes

TOP	*freesia, water lily, rose*
MIDDLE	*heliotrope, jasmine, orange blossom, narcissus*
LOWER	*sandalwood, amber, musk*

LALIQUE

*The house that revolutionized the way in which perfume is packaged
and sold*

PARENT COMPANY	*independent*
HEADQUARTERS	*Paris, France*
CURRENT PERFUMES	*Parfum Lalique, Nilang*

Like that of Baccarat, Lalique's fame in the perfume world is established around its bottles, but in recent years it has also issued some superb perfumes. René Lalique (1860–1945) founded a jewelry company in the Place Vendôme in Paris, France, in 1905, just as François Coty was founding his perfumery in the store next door. It was not long before Lalique was concentrating on glass design. He made his first perfume bottle for Coty, L'Effluert de Coty, in 1908.

It was the start of a long and lucrative association which revolutionized the way in which perfume was packaged and sold, and which arguably produced some of Lalique's finest bottle designs. Lalique indicated, quite simply, the best. Not only did it produce, as it still does, flacons for major perfume houses (such as D'Orsay, Fragonard, Houbigant, Guerlain, Lancôme, Molinard, Nina Ricci, Rochas, and Worth) but also bottles for the signature fragrances of many a couturier who wanted his scent in an outstandingly-crafted beautiful container.

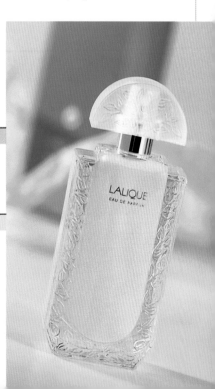

Parfum Lalique

LAUNCHED	*1992*
CREATOR	*Sophie Grosjman (IFF)*
CATEGORY	*floral*
FLACON	*Lalique*

notes

TOP	*gardenia, mandarin, blackberry*
MIDDLE	*peony, orange blossom, magnolia, rose, ylang-ylang*
LOWER	*sandalwood, cedar, oak moss, vanilla, musk, amber*

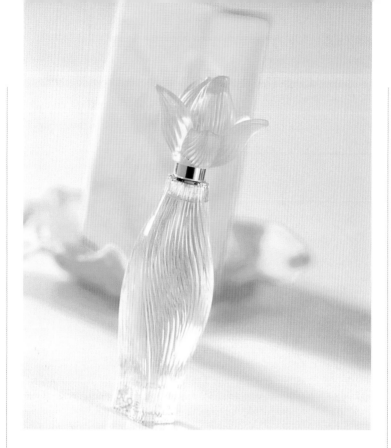

In the 1920s Lalique scent bottles were particularly noted for their Art Deco style. In postwar years Lalique has produced a decorative style which is distinctively its own. Remarkably both René's son Marc, who died in 1977, and then his granddaughter Marie-Claude Lalique, inherited his genius.

The company's first fragrance, Parfum Lalique, a fine floral scent, was launched in 1992. Apart from being in itself a high-quality perfume, it has the distinction of being reissued every year in a new limited-edition flacon. In 1994 the flacon was a design of nymphs and called Les Muses; for 1995 it was Jasmin, decorated with jasmine stems; in 1996 a naked figure, called Le Nu; and in 1997 Flacon Amour. On the bottle for Nilang, Lalique's second perfume, which was created by Gérard Anthony of Firmenich, the design is a lotus flower on a twisted stem.

Nilang

LAUNCHED *1995*

CREATOR *Gérard Anthony (Firmenich)*

CATEGORY *fresh aqua oriental and lotus*

FLACON *Lalique*

notes

TOP *water-jasmine, freesia, daffodil*

MIDDLE *lotus, bilberry*

LOWER *amber, vanilla, praline, sandalwood, musk*

LANCÔME

The brand with a rose, which for six decades has produced some of the world's most popular perfumes

PARENT COMPANY	*L'Oréal*
HEADQUARTERS	*Paris, France*
CURRENT PERFUMES	*Magie Noire, Trésor, Ô de Lancôme, Poême, Ô Oui*

Lancôme was founded in Paris, France, in 1935 by Armand Petitjean, a perfumer who had previously been managing-director of Coty, to produce fragrances and beauty products. He took its name from a romantic château in Touraine, France, called Château Lancosme and for his company's emblem he chose the rose.

In his first year Petitjean created five fragrances, starting with Conquête, together with a face powder and a lipstick, all manufactured at his own factory outside Paris and sold from his boutique in the Rue Faubourg St Honoré. New perfumes appeared steadily from then on, some 30 to date. By 1950 the company had well over 500 employees and in that year Petitjean bought land for a new headquarters and factory complex at Chevilly Larne, just south of Paris, which was finally occupied in 1964. Lancôme entered the British market in 1946 and opened in the USA a little later. Petitjean died in 1981.

These days Lancôme is noted both for its skincare products and as one of the world's leading perfume houses. Armand Petitjean personally created all the early fragrances, his greatest

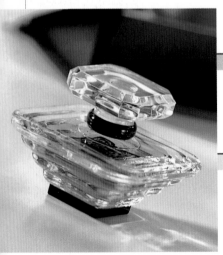

Trésor

LAUNCHED	*1990*
CREATOR	*Sophia Grosjman*
CATEGORY	*floral semi-oriental*
FLACON	*M. Swarowski (Style Marque)*

notes

TOP	*rose, lilac, lily of the valley*
MIDDLE	*iris, heliotrope*
LOWER	*sandalwood, musk, amber, vanilla, peach, apricot*

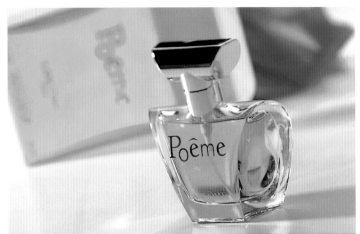

Poême

LANCHED *1995*
CREATOR *Jacques Cavallier
(Firmenich)*
CATEGORY *floral*
FLACON *Fabien Baron*

notes

*entirely floral—mimosa, jonquil,
freesia, rose, jasmine, daffodil,
vanilla flowers, datura, mecanopsis*

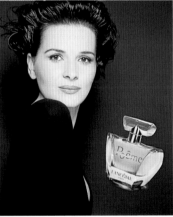

RIGHT:*Juliette Binoche—the face of
Lancôme in the 1990s.*

success being Magie, brought out in 1950 and still in demand 30 years later. It
was launched in a spectacular Lalique bottle (Lancôme had three other Lalique
flacons) and was later also sold in a bottle by Baccarat. Trésor was the first
Lancôme fragrance not created by Petitjean. Brought out in 1990, it was to
become their best seller of all time—a "hug me" perfume, according to its
creator, and also described as "a perfume with a history and a memory." The
brilliant flacon, like an inverted crystal pyramid, has added to its appeal. Poême,
which Lancôme brought out in 1995 using the face of Juliette Binoche, is a high-
quality fragrance composed entirely of floral notes. Lancôme's latest fragrance,
Ô Oui, a floral launched in 1998, aims to appeal to the younger woman, using
the face of the Belgian actress Marie Gillain, and its creator, Harry Fremont of
Firmenich, has described it as "a fragrance of pure air, a fruit sherbet with a dash
of vodka."

PARFUMS LANVIN

Creator of Arpège, the surviving reminder of this house's glorious past

PARENT COMPANY	*L'Oréal*
HEADQUARTERS	*Paris, France*
CURRENT PERFUME	*Arpège*

At the age of 16, in 1883, Jeanne Lanvin, the eldest in an impoverished family of 11 children, started making hats. Two years later she had her own business as a well-reputed milliner. She was soon married and almost as soon divorced, with a small daughter, Marie-Blanche, to bring up. She dressed Marie-Blanche in clothes she had made herself, and so good were they that her customers began to ask for similar dresses for their own daughters and then clothes for themselves as well.

So arose the concept of matching sets for mothers and daughters, which led to the famous Lanvin symbol, designed by the artist Iribe, showing her with Marie-Blanche in matching ball gowns. That symbol now appears on almost all Lanvin products.

Success as a couturier was quickly followed by success as a perfume house. In the early 1920s Jeanne Lanvin employed an elderly Russian perfumer, Madame Zen, to create fragrances to be sold with her clothes. The last of these was My Sin, which was widely acclaimed. She then decided to introduce a high-quality perfume to celebrate Marie-Blanche's 30th birthday. Two young perfumers, Paul Vacher and André Fraysse, were enrolled to work on this and in 1927, Arpège, one of the world's greatest perfumes, was launched. Arpège contains 62 ingredients representing an arpeggio of notes, for Marie-Blanche had become an accomplished musician. The flacon was an Art Deco design, a black ball with the Lanvin symbol and stopper, both in gold, but has undergone many revisions since.

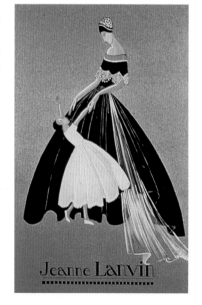

Jeanne Lanvin

RIGHT: *Iribe's original painting.*

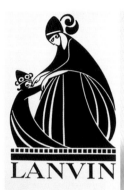

ABOVE: *The famous Lanvin symbol.*

Arpège

LAUNCHED **1927**
CREATOR **André Fraysse (with Paul Vacher)**
CATEGORY **floral aldehydic**
FLACON **Armand-Albert Rateau**

notes

TOP **bergamot, neroli, lily of the valley, orange blossom, honeysuckle, aldehydes**
MIDDLE **iris, ylang-ylang, jasmine, rose, camellia, lily of the valley**
LOWER **sandalwood, musk, patchouli, vetiver, vanilla, benzoin**

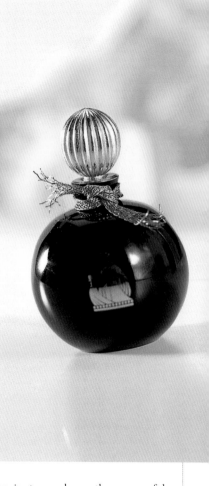

André Fraysse remained with Lanvin to produce other successful perfumes, notably Scandale, Rumeur, and, in 1937, Prétexte. At its peak it was said that the volume of flowers Lanvin used each year for its perfumes would fill the Arc de Triomphe. But fashions change and by the 1980s sales were falling, leading eventually to the acquisition of Lanvin by L'Oréal. Now only Arpège, reformulated in 1993 to appeal to a younger clientele, survives to remind us of a glorious past.

ESTÉE LAUDER

A dazzling range of modern and innovative fragrances

PARENT COMPANY	*independent*
HEADQUARTERS	*New York, USA*
CURRENT PERFUMES	*Youth Dew, Estée, Alliage, Private Collection, Cinnabar, White Linen, Beautiful, Knowing, Spellbound, Pleasures, White Linen Breeze, Dazzling Gold, Dazzling Silver*

Immediately after World War II a small company was set up in New York to sell four skincare products. Estée Lauder Companies Inc., founded by Estée and Joseph Lauder, is now one of the biggest skincare, make-up, and fragrance companies in the world and continues to expand. Members of the Estée Lauder family still play major roles in the group's operations. Other big-name companies form part of the group, as subsidiaries or licensees—famous names like Aramis, Clinique, Bobbi Brown, MAC, Origins, Prescriptives, Tommy Hilfiger, Jane, Donna Karan, and Aveda.

The Estée Lauder company has some 12,000 employees; and outside of the USA it manufactures its cosmetic products in Australia, Belgium, Canada, England, and Switzerland.

The fragrance side of the Estée Lauder business has itself been enormous, right from the time in

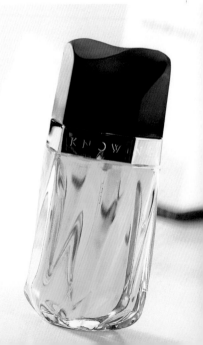

Knowing

LAUNCHED *1988*
CREATOR *Firmenich perfumers*
CATEGORY *floral chypre*
FLACON *Ira Levy*

notes

TOP *rose, pittosporum, mimosa, tuberose, davana, plum, melon*

MIDDLE *jasmine, lily of the valley, patchouli, orris, bay*

LOWER *oak moss, amber, sandalwood, vetiver, musk*

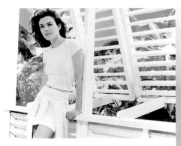

ABOVE: *Advertisement for White Linen Breeze.*

Pleasures

LAUNCHED **1995**
CREATOR **Firmenich perfumers**
CATEGORY **floral**
FLACON **Ateliers Dinand**

notes

TOP **lily, violet leaf**
MIDDLE **lilac, peony, pink, jasmine, rose, karo-karundi, baie rose**
LOWER **sandalwood, patchouli**

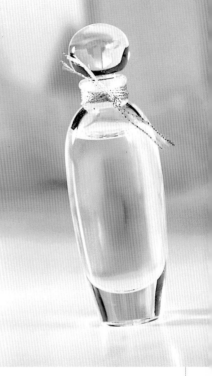

1953 when she launched Youth Dew, which bridged the gap between bath oil and fragrance with a perfume that has become an innovative classic. Estée followed in 1968. Then the spicy green and woody Alliage, followed by Private Collection, with its floral, woody notes, the crisp oriental Cinnabar, and the clean, fresh, springlike White Linen, all of these fragrances made their mark in the 1970s, contained by this time in flacons shaped by Ira Levy, Estée Lauder's own bottle designer.

In 1986 came Beautiful, with its bridal-bouquet image in a composition containing no fewer than 19 different flower scents, and then Knowing (1988), a modern chypre for women who knew what they were about. "It's a fragrance for the twentieth century," Estée Lauder claimed, "because it is a fragrance ahead of its time for a woman in control of her life, her present and her future." But Knowing also brought something new into perfumery, an elusive fragrance which Estée Lauder had herself noticed in her garden in the South of France and which was found to be pittosporum, then used in a perfume for the first time.

In the 1990s five major launches have already taken place, starting with Spellbound in 1992, the floriental fragrance "which will leave him mesmerized." Pleasures arrived in 1995, designed to evoke the clarity of fragrance coming

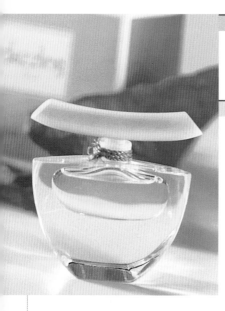

Dazzling Gold

LAUNCHED *1998*
CREATOR *Evelyn Lauder*
CATEGORY *floral*
FLACON *Ira Levy*

notes

TOP *passion flower, fig*
MIDDLE *orchid, lily, plumiera*
LOWER *sandalwood, amber,*
vanilla

from flowers covered with rain; it brought with it two unusual new ingredients—Baie Rose, a spice from Réunion Island, and Karo Karundi, from the flowers of a West African shrub—and they help to provide a surprising peppery note with the sensuous floral tones. Pleasures may also be noted as the first Estée Lauder fragrance fronted by Elizabeth Hurley.

A year later White Linen Breeze followed, bringing the line of Estée Lauder perfumes up to date with light ozonic notes (the scent of the ocean and seashore) first developed by Dior in Dune five years earlier. It is a perfume designed to go with relaxed sunny afternoons, cool breezes, and sparkling water.

Latest in the Estée Lauder series is Dazzling, which promotes the notion of providing two complementary yet contradictory perfumes together. Dazzling Gold is in the romantic, classic style and Dazzling Silver is made for more spirited occasions. Both come in full *parfum* concentration.

Dazzling Silver

LAUNCHED *1998*
CREATOR *Evelyn Lauder*
CATEGORY *floral*
FLACON *Ira Levy*

notes

TOP *lily, sunshine flower,*
lotus, orchid, vanilla
MIDDLE *orchid, passion flower,*
rose
LOWER *magnolia wood, ginger*
lily

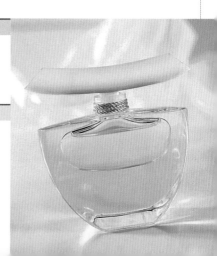

RALPH LAUREN

An American in Paris, creator of fragrances on sporting themes

PARENT COMPANY	*L'Oréal*
HEADQUARTERS	*New York, USA*
CURRENT PERFUMES	*Lauren, Safari, Polo Sport Woman, Romance*

Men's neckties were the first articles that Ralph Lauren started to design. So good was he at it that he became famous for them. But it was not long before he was designing other things as well. By 1989 the man born in New York 50 years before was the head of what had become a very large fashion empire, with over 130 stores spread all over the world.

Ralph Lauren designed and produced all sorts of clothing, together with footwear, jewelry, luggage, and furniture, and from 1978 he entered the world of fragrances. He has the distinction of being the first American designer to open premises in Paris.

Lauren's first perfume for women was a fruity-fresh floral called Lauren, in a cube-shaped bottle designed by Barnard Kotyuk. He introduced this at the same time as Polo for Men. Always following the theme of sport, athletics, and the outdoor life, he next produced, in 1990, the highly esteemed Safari, which won a FiFi award as most successful women's fragrance (together with a second such award

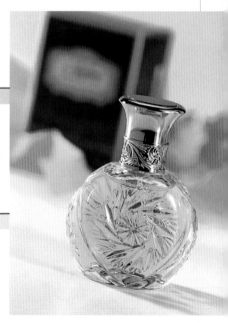

Safari

LAUNCHED	*1990*
CREATOR	*Dominique Ropion (Roure, later with Florasynth, now part of Haarmann & Reimer)*
CATEGORY	*floral green*
FLACON	*Ben Kotyuk*

notes

TOP	*tagette, jonquil, mandarin*
MIDDLE	*narcissus, broom, rose, orange blossom*
LOWER	*sandalwood, amber, patchouli*

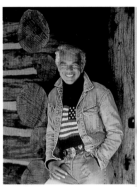

ABOVE: *Ralph Lauren.*

Polo Sport Woman

LAUNCHED *1996*
CREATOR *Jim Krivda (Mane)*
CATEGORY *"cool, translucent, floral"*
FLACON *Richard Lavigne*

notes

TOP *water mint, penny royal, citrus, orange flower, eucalyptus, melon*
MIDDLE *poppy, freesia, lily, ylang-ylang, nutmeg, ginger*
LOWER *sandalwood, cedar, musk, oak, ebony*

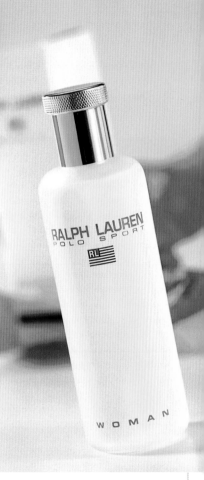

for its TV advertising). Its creator, Dominique Ropion, also created Ysatis and Amarige. Safari has been described as having a feminine, out-of-Africa feel, which is emphasized by its heavy, sophisticated, decanter-shaped flacon of cut glass, with a silvery orb-shaped stopper stamped with the Lauren monogram and contained in a mock-crocodile-skin box. The whole image is of big-game hunting in a bygone era.

In 1996 Ralph Lauren launched Polo Sport Woman, a fragrance designed for "the woman who regards fitness as the ultimate beauty tool." It is made only up to *eau de toilette* concentration and, in accordance with current trends for such fragrances, contains an element of skincare oils among its ingredients. It also includes an interesting formulation based on sea rocket, sea kelp, sea fennel, and algae. Romance was launched in the USA at the end of 1998.

PARFUMS LELONG

The "first gentleman of fashion" and creator of flacons that are collectors' items

PARENT COMPANY	*Arnold & Lucy Neis*
HEADQUARTERS	*New York, USA*
CURRENT PERFUMES	*Indiscret*

The return in 1998 of Lucien Lelong's distinguished bestseller Indiscret is much to be welcomed, for it reminds us not only of an important perfume house that had disappeared but also of one of France's major couturiers. Lelong (1889–1958), holder of the Croix de Guerre, opened his fashion house in 1919 and was highly successful.

Known as "the first gentleman of fashion," he designed for some of the greatest beauties of the 1930s and established the idea that elegant dresses could be made and sold at affordable prices for the less wealthy. During World War II he ran a couture-house organization which frustrated all German attempts to move the fashion industry to Berlin.

After the war he perceived the talents of designers such as Balmain, Dior, and Givenchy, all of whom trained with him. But in 1948 he had to give up designing for health reasons. He opened Parfums Lelong in 1924 and designed many of the 50 Lelong flacons himself, all now prized collectors' pieces. The Indiscret bottle was made to look like folds of silk. Further perfumes are expected from Parfums Lelong.

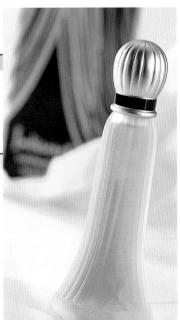

Indiscret

LAUNCHED	*1936, relaunched 1997*
CREATOR	*Mane perfumers (for relaunch)*
CATEGORY	*floral fruity*
FLACON	*Lelong, Marc Rosen*

notes

TOP	*mandarin, orange flower, bergamot, orchid, neroli*
MIDDLE	*iris, galbanum, tuberose, jasmine, ylang-ylang*
LOWER	*oak moss, vetivert, guaiac, patchouli, sandalwood*

PARFUMS LOLITA LEMPICKA

A fragrance of unusual composition, the winner of three major fragrance awards

PARENT COMPANY	*Pacific Corporation*
HEADQUARTERS	*Paris, France*
CURRENT PERFUME	*Lolita Lempicka*

Parfums Lolita Lempicka is the fragrance division of the Paris fashion business run by the prominent designer of this name, and its first perfume—her debut fragrance—is also named after her. The parent company is Korean.

Lolita Lempicka, the perfume, was launched in 1997 (in the UK not until late 1998) and has had quite an impact already, winning the 1998 French FiFi award for best feminine fragrance and then, in June 1998, the award for best European feminine fragrance at the FiFi main award ceremony in New York. In addition, it was voted best 1997 fragrance by the influential French trade journal *Cosmétique News*, which also gave it two awards for its advertising. This is a considerable record.

It is of unusual composition, having been built up as two fragrances in one, each with its own top, middle, and lower notes—the first a floral, the second an innovative licorice fragrance. It is also unusual in being made solely at *eau de parfum* concentration.

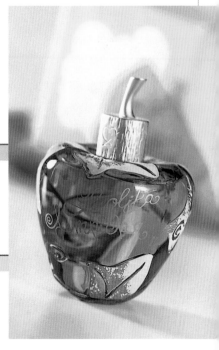

Lolita Lempicka

LAUNCHED	*1997*
CREATOR	*Annick Ménardeau (Firmenich)*
CATEGORY	*floral semi-oriental*
FLACON	*Alain de Mourges and Pochet et du Courval*

notes

TOP	*aniseed, ivy*
MIDDLE	*violet, iris, Amarena cherry*
LOWER	*vanilla, praline, vetiver, tonka, musk*

PARFUMS LOEWE

Part of an exclusive group of perfume houses, with stores from East to West

PARENT COMPANY	*Louis Vuitton, Moët, Hennessy (LVMH)*
HEADQUARTERS	*Madrid, Spain*
CURRENT PERFUMES	*Aire Loewe, Gala Loewe*

Aire Loewe

LAUNCHED	*1992*
CREATORS	*Quest perfumers*
CATEGORY	*fresh floral*
FLACON	*in-house*

notes

TOP	*petitgrain, mandarin, lemon, tagette, galbanum*
MIDDLE	*jasmine, ylang-ylang, iris, lily of the valley, frankincense, amber*
LOWER	*sandalwood, vetiver, musk*

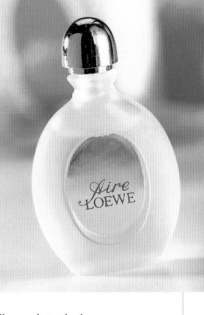

Despite its name, the Loewe (pronounced "Lo-ay-vay") company has a Spanish origin, being founded in Madrid, and for its first 120 years it had nothing to do with perfume. The founder was a German who had emigrated to Spain and who, in 1846, set up a store selling exclusive leatherware.

His business was very successful and the company expanded with equal success into fashion and ready-to-wear clothing. It now has stores all over Spain and in London, Paris, New York, Mexico, Portugal, Arabia, and the Far East (including 19 in Japan), and is a part of the exclusive LVMH Group together with Dior, Guerlain, Givenchy, and others.

Loewe's perfume division, Parfums Loewe, was inaugurated in 1976 with the launch of the perfume Loewe, but no further fragrances for women were issued until Aire Loewe in 1992. At the same time Loewe also introduced Gala Loewe, which came in a notable blue and gold bottle and cap in a design inspired by the Infanta's dress in Velasquez' famous painting *Las Meninas*.

JO MALONE

Creator of a wide range of products using high-quality natural materials

PARENT COMPANY	*independent*
HEADQUARTERS	*London, England*
CURRENT PERFUMES	*Lime, Basil & Mandarin, Wild Muguet, Gardenia, Tuberose, Verbena of Provence, Fleurs de la Forêt, and many others*

Jo Malone recollects pushing rose petals into miniature bottles in early childhood. The daughter of professional parents living in London's prestigious Chelsea district (her father was an architect, her mother a beautician), she has been fascinated by oils and fragrances all her life, and started her career giving facial massages and mixing ingredients for her special skin tonics.

She married Gary Willcox in 1983 and he became her business partner. In 1994 a store was opened in London's Walton Street designed to create the atmosphere of an early French perfumer's studio. The business has never looked back. New boutiques have opened in London, at Bergdorf Goodman's in New York, at Joseph's in Paris, and elsewhere.

New fragrance undertakings have been launched: Scent an Event helps commercial companies to perfume their fashion shows and sales conferences—she has even perfumed the Royal Albert Hall in London. Sent a Scent delivers personalized fragrance gifts. Fragrance Combining provides unique scents made to clients' own specifications. She has a wide range of products, using high-quality natural materials at up to *cologne* concentration. Jo Malone's signature perfume is Lime, Basil & Mandarin.

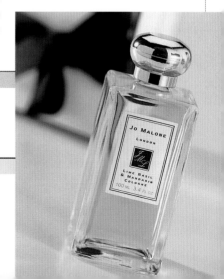

Lime, Basil & Mandarin

LAUNCHED	*1991*
CREATOR	*Jo Malone*
CATEGORY	*hesperidic*
FLACON	*n/a*

notes

TOP	*mandarin, lime*
MIDDLE	*jasmine, lilac, basil, white thyme*
LOWER	*woody, vetiver*

NICOLE MILLER

The dress designer of international repute, with an "explosive" signature perfume

PARENT COMPANY	*independent*
HEADQUARTERS	*New York, USA*
CURRENT PERFUMES	*Nicole Miller*

Accidents can sometimes lead to unexpected successes, as was the case with the New York dress designer Nicole Miller. As head designer for P.J. Walsh, she established a high reputation for the quality of her artwork on printed fabrics. In 1982 she bought up the company with a partner, Bud Konheim, and gave it her name, subsequently opening a store in Madison Avenue where she could sell her silhouette fashions.

By error some ties were made from a discarded dress print. The Metropolitan Opera Gift Shop bought them and ordered hundreds more. New prints were added and the notion of selling small items for men from a women's boutique took off. She is now an established international dress designer and owns stores and boutiques throughout the USA and in many other countries. It seemed natural for a signature perfume to follow. Nicole Miller, described as "an explosive aura-floral perfume, young, fun, and exciting," comes in a bottle resembling a leather pouch tied round with gold cord.

Nicole Miller

LAUNCHED	*1993*
CREATOR	*Xavier Renard (Givaudan-Roure)*
CATEGORY	*floral fruity oriental*
FLACON	*Pierre Dinand*

notes

TOP	*mandarin, cyclamen, freesia, ylang-ylang, peach*
MIDDLE	*rose, jasmine, tuberose, clove, orange flower, heliotrope*
LOWER	*sandalwood, vanilla, musk, amber, tonka, opopanax*

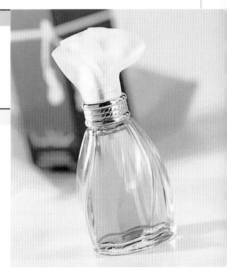

ISSEY MIYAKE

*The design genius who created the highly successful fragrance,
Eau d'Issey*

PARENT COMPANY	*Shiseido*
HEADQUARTERS	*Paris, France, and Tokyo, Japan*
CURRENT PERFUMES	*L'Eau d'Issey, Le Feu d'Issey*

It is difficult to fathom out a designer like Issey Miyake. He is Japanese, but learned his profession as a fashion designer in Paris, working initially under Guy Laroche and Hubert de Givenchy. He is a minimalist, yet full of design ideas which are really highly complicated.

He is certainly unusual and mysterious. When asked to design costumes for a 1991 ballet in Frankfurt with a cast of 40, he was given carte blanche and made 400 of them. Miyake presented his first clothes collection in Paris in 1973, after creating the Miyake Design Studio there three years earlier.

He has produced just one full perfume for women, the very successful Eau d'Issey, together with the floral-spicy-woody fragrance Le Feu d'Issey, which was launched as an *eau de toilette* at the end of 1998. His fragrance business now belongs to the huge Japanese company Shiseido, giving his fragrances both the substantial backing needed to compete in the international market and assistance from Shiseido's eminent design director, Fabien Baron.

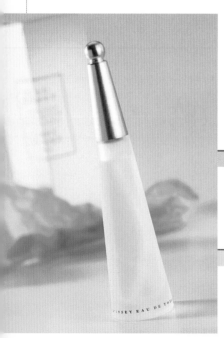

L'Eau d'Issey

LAUNCHED	*1991*
CREATOR	*Jacques Cavallier (Firmenich)*
CATEGORY	*floral woody*
FLACON	*Alain de Morgues*

notes

TOP	*freesia, rose, cyclamen, lotus*
MIDDLE	*peony, lily, carnation*
LOWER	*tuberose, osmanthus, musk*

MOLINARD

The perfume house with a long history, particularly noted for its famous Lalique flacons

PARENT COMPANY	*independent*
HEADQUARTERS	*Paris, France*
CURRENT PERFUMES	*Habanita, Molinard de Molinard, Les Senteurs (series), Les Femmes (series), Eau Fraîche, Eau de Cologne France*

Even before the French Revolution it used to be said that half of Europe extracted its essences from Grasse. Grasse had long been a leather-making center and, when a fashion arose for scented gloves, the tanners of Grasse exercised their royally bestowed right to make perfume for their finely produced apparel. It marked the foundation of Grasse as the perfume capital of the world.

In 1849 one Molinard Jeune came to Grasse to sell his "perfumed water" from a small store. Business prospered and by the end of the century his company had built its own distillery. Molinard had a prestigious clientele, including Queen Victoria of England, who visited Grasse, and around the end of the century it built a center in Grasse to receive the customers who wintered on the Riviera.

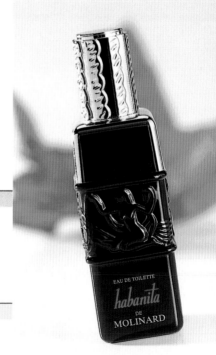

Habanita

LAUNCHED	*1924, relaunched 1988*
CREATORS	*Molinard perfumers / 1988 Roure perfumers*
CATEGORY	*oriental*
FLACON	*Lalique*

notes

TOP	*bergamot, peach*
MIDDLE	*rose, ylang-ylang*
LOWER	*vanilla, leather*

Molinard de Molinard

LAUNCHED	*1980*
CREATOR	*Molinard perfumers*
CATEGORY	*fruity green floral*
FLACON	*Lalique*

notes

TOP	*galbanum, blackcurrant*
MIDDLE	*jasmine, rose, narcissus, ylang-ylang, lily of the valley*
LOWER	*labdanum, frankincense, amber, musk, vetiver*

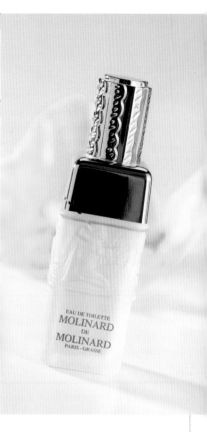

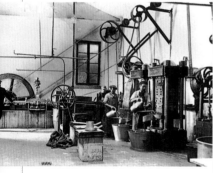

ABOVE: *Molinard workers making pomade, c. 1920.*

Today this salon, still owned by Molinard, is a splendid museum, open to the public, showing a collection of antique furniture and, more especially, bottles, documents, machinery, and other objects to do with perfumery. Molinard had moved its headquarters to Paris by 1920, becoming known as Le Société Bénard et Honorat after its then owners, but reverted to the name Molinard in 1938.

Over its long history there have, of course, been very many Molinard perfumes produced, but perhaps the fragrance that has made the most impact in the perfume world was Habanita, first launched in 1924. It is one of several perfumes which Molinard has presented in a famous flacon designed by Lalique known to collectors as Beauty, featuring a relief decoration of water nymphs. Other Lalique flacons have also been used by Molinard, most famous being Le Baiser du Faune, which won a medal in New York in the 1932 Exhibition as the most beautiful flacon in the world. Besides Habanita, Molinard now has another bestselling fragrance, Molinard de Molinard, a rich floral containing over 600 ingredients.

PARFUMS MONTANA

Creator of the fragrance that comes in an award-winning bottle of outstanding design

PARENT COMPANY	*Clarins*
HEADQUARTERS	*Paris, France*
CURRENT PERFUMES	*Parfum de Peau, Parfum d'Elle, Just Me*

Claude Montana has been a prominent fashion designer in Paris since 1976 and first made his name for his work in leather. He set up his own company in 1979 and was the first designer to win the Paris fashion industry's Gold Award in two consecutive years. His business was acquired by Clarins, for whom he now designs, in 1995.

Montana founded Parfums Montana with the launch of his first fragrance in 1986. At first called Montana, it is now named Parfum de Peau and is described as an *avant-garde* chypre. It comes in a flacon of outstanding design, with spiral layers of frosted glass recalling a woman's body in motion, which won the French glass industry's award for the outstanding bottle of the year.

In 1989 Montana produced another well-received perfume, the floriental Parfum d'Elle, in a bottle shaped like a conch shell with similar frosted-glass layers, again designed by Serge Mansau. Just Me was launched in 1997 (not in the UK).

Parfum de Peau

LAUNCHED	*1986*
CREATOR	*Jean Guichard (Roure)—reformulated 1997 by Edouard Fléchier (Givaudan-Roure)*
CATEGORY	*chypre*
FLACON	*Serge Mansau*

notes

TOP	*marigold, ginger, pepper, blackcurrant buds, orange flower*
MIDDLE	*jasmine, rose, narcissus, patchouli*
LOWER	*ambrein, musk, frankincense, leather*

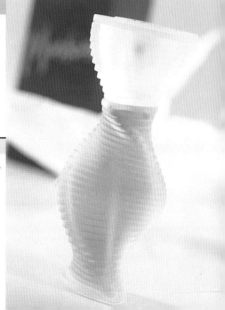

POPY MORENI

The fashion designer whose signature perfume evokes memories of her childhood

PARENT COMPANY	*Fragrance Plus*
HEADQUARTERS	*Paris, France*
CURRENT PERFUMES	*Popy Moreni, Popy Moreni de Fête*

The fashion designer Popy Moreni is Italian by birth but has lived in France for over 40 years and is now based in a small store in the Place des Vosges in Paris. Her father was an artist and her mother a sculptress.

After studying at the Turin Fashion Institute, she found work as an adviser on design to companies involved in textiles, clothing, and interior decoration, and her fashions reflect the disciplines of those days, with a firm eye to balance, quality, and detail. She herself dresses austerely in black and white, but her designs blend a riot of color, with much use of ruffs and scarves.

Moreni's signature perfume, named after her, brings out memories of her childhood, like talcum powder and garden flowers, and the packaging reflects her present-day life, with a ruff, a dress, a needle, and a cone-shaped hat in the bottle design and black and white cubes on the box. In 1997 it won the *Cosmétique News* award for the best perfume of the year. She has now launched a second perfume, called Popy Moreni de Fête.

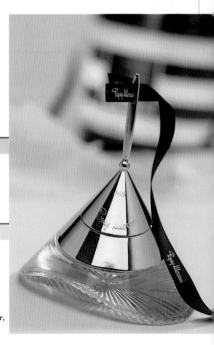

Popy Moreni

LAUNCHED	*1996*
CREATOR	*Martin Gras (Dragoco)*
CATEGORY	*powdery floral*
FLACON	*Thierry de Bashmakoff*

notes

TOP	*ylang-ylang, bergamot, geranium, coffee*
MIDDLE	*mimosa, cilantro, orange blossom, heliotrope, broom*
LOWER	*styrax, patchouli, vetiver, sandalwood, amber*

THIERRY MUGLER

Creator of the angelic fragrance that conjures memories of fairgrounds and cotton candy

PARENT COMPANY	*Clarins*
HEADQUARTERS	*Paris, France*
CURRENT PERFUMES	*Angel, Angel Innocent*

A citizen of Strasbourg, Thierry Mugler joined the *corps de ballet* of the Opera of the Rhine at the age of 14 and started to wear clothes of his own design and making. In Paris, age 20, he was window designer for a trendy boutique and a freelance stylist for various fashion houses. He presented his first collection in 1973, which was well received, and subsequently started up the fashion house that bears his name.

His style is always *avant-garde* and angels are a recurring theme, symbolizing the dualities he sees in women—soft yet strong, innocent yet seductive. His first perfume, Angel, was designed to be quite different from others of that time—essentially it should not fade away when fashions changed. The bottle was to be based on a star of blue-tinged crystal, another of Mugler's concepts, but for contrast with the coldness of the glass the perfume was to be warm and earthy, reminiscent of childhood experiences of fairgrounds, cotton candy, and chocolate mixed with an elixir of fruit and caramel. It took 18 months to devise this complicated fragrance, which is issued in up to *eau de parfum* concentration.

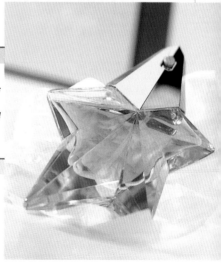

Angel

LAUNCHED	*1994*
CREATORS	*Olivier Cresp and Yves de Chirin (Quest)*
CATEGORY	*oriental fruity gourmand*
FLACON	*Thierry Mugler with Brosse*

notes

TOP	*bergamot, jasmine*
MIDDLE	*red berries, dewberry, honey*
LOWER	*patchouli, vanilla, coumarin, chocolate, caramel*

PARFUMS DE NICOLAÏ

Fragrances that are simple but of high quality, using natural ingredients

PARENT COMPANY	*independent*
HEADQUARTERS	*Paris, France*
CURRENT PERFUMES	*Rose Pivoine, Eau d'Été, Juste un Rêve, Vanilla Tonka, Sacrebleu, Mimosaïque, Eau de Cheverny*

As a granddaughter of the man who founded Guerlain, Patricia de Nicolaï could be expected to know a lot about scent. Her background proves that she does. After graduating in 1980 from the French School of Perfumery and working with a perfume-creation company, she and her husband, Jean-Louis Michau, set up their own company, Parfums de Nicolaï, in 1989.

Her first perfume, called Number One, won her that year's coveted award for Best International Perfumer from La Société Technique des Parfumeurs; she was the first woman perfumer to achieve this. She has also devised and sells a high-tech "diffuser" that will perfume a house and at the same time destroy any bad smells in it. She now lives in London, but her factory is near Orléans, in France. The Nicolaï fragrances are simple but are of a very high quality and are very sophisticated. The scents are made using natural ingredients.

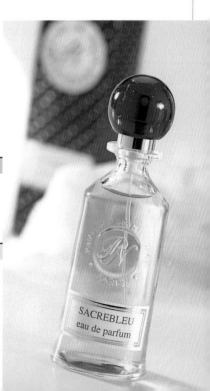

Sacrebleu

LAUNCHED	*1993*
CREATOR	*Patricia de Nicolaï*
CATEGORY	*floral oriental*
FLACON	*in-house*

notes

TOP	*blackcurrant buds, raspberry, apricot*
MIDDLE	*jasmine, cinnamon, clove-pink*
LOWER	*vanilla, civet, castoreum*

RIFAT OZBEK

A signature perfume in a minaret flacon, from an award-winning designer of fashion

PARENT COMPANY	*Aeffe Spa*
HEADQUARTERS	*London, England*
CURRENT PERFUMES	*Ozbek*

Ozbek

LAUNCHED	*1995*
CREATOR	*n/a*
CATEGORY	*floral*
FLACON	*Rifat Ozbek*

notes

TOP	*rosewood, freesia, peach*
MIDDLE	*pittosporum, jasmine, ylang-ylang, hyacinth*
LOWER	*musk, honey*

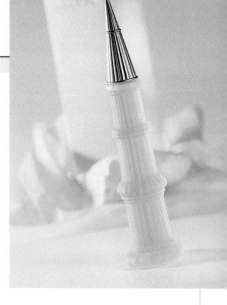

This highly rated fashion designer grew up in Istanbul, where he was born, and moved to London with the intention of studying architecture. Having realized that his real interest was fashion, he enrolled at the St Martin's School of Art, graduating with honors, and formed his own company under the Ozbek label in 1984.

He now has a distinguished reputation worldwide and a considerable following, although he shrinks from personal publicity, preferring a reserved private life with a simple lifestyle.

His collections reflect contemporary themes in a fusing of ethnic elements and modern culture and an eclectic mix of colors and textures. He has twice been the recipient of the British Fashion Council's Designer of the Year award. His company is tied in financially with an Italian group.

Rifat Ozbek launched his signature perfume, Ozbek, in 1995 with a full line, but he has not followed it with any other fragrance. The flacon is splendid and most unusual, a representation of a Turkish minaret.

JEAN PATOU

The great fashion innovator who produced Joy, "the costliest perfume in the world"

PARENT COMPANY	*independent*
HEADQUARTERS	*Paris, France*
CURRENT PERFUMES	*Joy, 1000 (Mille), Eau de Patou, Ma Liberté, Sublime, Ma Collection series (Amour-Amour, Que Sais-Je?, Adieu Sagesse, Chaldée, Moment Suprême, Cocktail, Divine Folie, Normandie, Vacances, Colony, L'Heure Attendue, Câline), Patou Forever*

Jean Patou was a great innovator. Born the son of a Normandy tanner in 1887, he moved to Paris, France, in 1910, served in the trenches during World War I, founded his fashion and perfume house in 1919, and died in 1936 aged 49. He was essentially a man of the 1920s and 1930s and he seems to have come into the fashion world quite suddenly, for we hear little of him until he presented his first collection in 1919.

That was a great success and fame followed quickly. In a very short time he was opening an office in New York.

Patou gave women a new sense of freedom in their clothing while retaining their femininity. He diversified into sportswear (making Susanne Lenglen the first designer tennis shorts, for example),

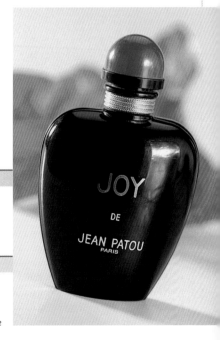

Joy

LAUNCHED	*1930*
CREATOR	*Henri Alméras*
CATEGORY	*floral*
FLACON	*Louis Süe*

notes

TOP	*rose, tuberose, ylang-ylang*
MIDDLE	*rose, jasmine*
LOWER	*sandalwood, musk, civet*

originated jersey cardigans and knitted bathing suits, introduced complementary accessories for his clothes, put his monogram on them where it showed, produced the first suntan lotion. Elsa Maxwell once said he had more sex appeal than any other man she knew. But he could also be reckless, gambled, and liked fast cars, boats, and women.

After Patou's death his brother-in-law and closest friend, Raymond Barbas, continued to run the company in the same style and spirit, adding a wide range of what Patou had described as "little nothings"—jewelry, scarves, sunglasses, and so on. The company remains under family control, with Jean de Moüy, Patou's greatnephew, the present chairman.

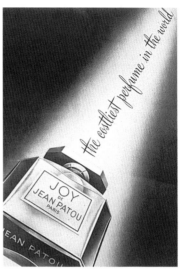

ABOVE: *Sales of Joy confirmed that no price is too high for perfume.*

Patou introduced his first three perfumes together in 1925—Amour-Amour, Que Sais-Je?, and Adieu Sagesse. To create them he employed Henri Alméras, already well known for his perfumes for Paul Poiret's company Rosine. Moment Suprême followed in 1929 and the next year saw Joy, called "the costliest perfume in the world." Oddly, Joy immediately followed the Wall Street crash.

Jean Patou wanted to send a gift to his many regular international clients who he knew would be unable to visit Paris that year. He asked Alméras to create something very strong and simple, and it was to be made regardless of the cost of the ingredients. It is the quality of the rose and jasmine used which makes Joy so special; one ounce, it is said, requires over 10,000 jasmine flowers and 28 dozen roses.

The flacon was designed to classical proportions by Louis Süe, but another was later inspired by one of Patou's own antique Chinese snuff bottles and a third was produced by Baccarat.

Many other perfumes followed this unique fragrance. These scents were created for the company by its own perfumer in its own factory at Levallois-Perret. Among them may be noted L'Heure Attendue, Patou's celebration of the end of the war. The Patou perfumer is now Jean Kerleo, who succeeded Alméras after a long period with Helena Rubinstein, and who has created all Patou fragrances since 1969, including 1000 (Mille) and its latest, the intensely feminine Sublime. In 1984 a series of 12 earlier perfumes were reissued together as a group called Ma Collection.

PENHALIGON'S

The company that was transformed into a distinguished perfume house, producing high-quality fragrances

PARENT COMPANY	*independent*
HEADQUARTERS	*London, England*
CURRENT PERFUMES	*Lily of the Valley, Victorian Posy, Bluebell, Cornubia, Ormolu, Elizabethan Rose, Violetta, Love Potion No. 9*

William Penhaligon was a barber from the county of Cornwall in England who found his way to London, where he set up a perfume shop in Jermyn Street in 1870. The business flourished while he was running it, but fell apart after his death and remained at a very low ebb until 1975.

In that year it was revived by a remarkable woman, Sheila Pickles, who started to transform it into a distinguished perfume house producing a wide range of high-quality, single-note fragrances in lines up to *extrait* concentration, together with items such as silver-topped crystal flacons, perfume pens, scented candles, bath oils, body lotions, and other toiletry articles. The company is now one of the foremost of its type and has eight branches in London, together with others in France and the USA.

In the past Penhaligon's has had clients such as Sir Winston Churchill and today it holds royal warrants to supply both the Duke of Edinburgh and the Prince of Wales.

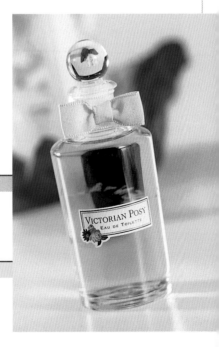

Victorian Posy

LAUNCHED	*1979*
CREATOR	*n/a*
CATEGORY	*floral*
FLACON	*n/a*

notes

LINEAR *wild rose, winter jasmine, lily of the valley, camomile, oak moss*

LA PERLA

Intimate, seductive fragrances from the family-run Italian fashion house

PARENT COMPANY	*Henkel KGAA of Düsseldorf*
HEADQUARTERS	*Bologna, Italy*
CURRENT PERFUMES	*La Perla, Io La Perla, Parfum Privé*

La Perla is an Italian fashion group which was founded in Bologna in northern Italy by Ada Masotti in 1954. Silk textiles have been a traditional product of Bologna since the sixteenth century, so Ada Masotti's small workshop making high-quality lingerie fitted happily into its surroundings and flourished. The company has become one of the largest fashion houses in Italy, employing over 2,000 people.

It opened its first overseas store in Madison Avenue, New York, in 1994 and now has stores and boutiques in Paris, London, and elsewhere, selling lingerie, swimming costumes, and other clothing. Although now owned by a large German company, it remains a family-run business under Ada's son Alberto Masotti, who was formerly a doctor.

La Perla introduced their first fragrance, La Perla, in 1986. They wanted something intimate, seductive, and luxurious and IFF perfumers found this for them with an interesting floral chypre perfume. A top note of flowers and citrus leads into a very floral heart tinged with spices and some sensual base notes. Io La Perla followed in 1995 in a more woody and fruity format, created by Daniella Roche of Givaudan-Roure.

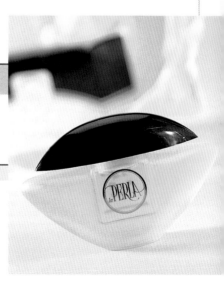

La Perla
(also called La Perla Bodysilk)

LAUNCHED	*1995*
CREATORS	*IFF perfumers*
CATEGORY	*floral chypre*
FLACON	*Pierre Dinand*

notes

TOP	*carnation, freesia, osmanthus, mandarin*
MIDDLE	*jasmine, rose, cilantro, pepper, cardamom*
LOWER	*patchouli, oak moss, musk*

PARFUMS PALOMA PICASSO

Daughter of the famous Pablo, and winner of two FiFi awards for
Mon Parfum

PARENT COMPANY	*L'Oréal*
HEADQUARTERS	*Paris, France*
CURRENT PERFUMES	*Mon Parfum, Tentations*

From the angle of perfume the important point about Paloma Picasso is that her mother, Françoise Gilot, was the daughter of Emile Gilot, a perfumer who worked in Grasse, France. As a child Paloma was fascinated by the scents of his workshop and the whole art of perfumery which she encountered there. Perfume was thus a part of her life since childhood.

But the influence of her famous father, Pablo Picasso, also had a bearing. As befits the daughter of a great artist, she also has a remarkable, original, and eclectic sense of design, form, and color, and that shows itself in the bottles and packaging she chooses for her perfumes.

Paloma, named after the dove that her father designed as a symbol for the World Peace Conference, started her working life in 1971 designing jewelry for Zolotas, a Greek company. In 1980 she joined the élite Tiffany company in New

Mon Parfum

LAUNCHED	*1984*
CREATORS	*perfumers of Créations Aromatiques*
CATEGORY	*chypre*
FLACON	*Paloma Picasso with Bernard Kotyuk*

notes

TOP	*lemon, bergamot, angelica, hyacinth, ylang-ylang*
MIDDLE	*rose, jasmine, mimosa, cilantro*
LOWER	*oak moss, iris, sandalwood, patchouli, amber, musk, honey*

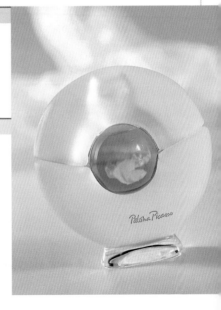

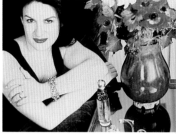

ABOVE: *Paloma Picasso.*

Tentations

LAUNCHED *1997*
CREATORS *perfumers of IFF*
CATEGORY *spicy woody floriental*
FLACON *Paloma Picasso*

notes

TOP *vine flower*
MIDDLE *rose, jasmine, pepper,*
spicy notes
LOWER *frankincense, myrrh,*
cedar

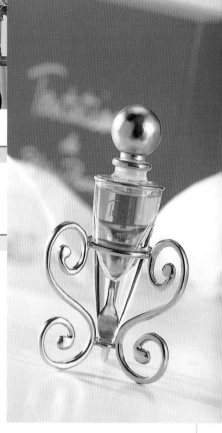

York, where her unique design style, with bold shapes and unexpected combinations, quickly made its mark.

She now has her own business, extending from jewelry to scarves, purses, sunglasses, and many other fashion accessories, and she has designed collections of china, crystal, silver, and tiles for Villeroy & Boch as well as fabric and wall coverings for Motif.

Her taste is daring and unconventional and she takes a lively interest in every stage in the production of what she has designed. In 1980 she was elected onto the short list of "the most elegant women in the world" and in 1983 she won that title.

Paloma Picasso's first perfume was Mon Parfum (also called Paloma Picasso), which was launched in 1984 (1985 in Europe) and attracted considerable attention, winning two FiFi awards. The flacon followed one of her favorite themes, a circle within a circle, and was inspired by her design for an earring she had done for Tiffany. Since 1991 a sample of this bottle has been on permanent display in the Musée des Arts Decoratifs in Paris.

PARFUMS ROBERT PIGUET

*Creators of Fracas—a fragrance that's eccentric, provocative,
revolutionary, and a little wild*

PARENT COMPANY	*Fashion Fragrances*
HEADQUARTERS	*New Jersey, USA*
CURRENT PERFUMES	*Fracas*

Robert Piguet (1901–1953) formed his fashion company in 1928 and was to become one of the leading *haute couture* designers in Paris. Christian Dior, Hugh de Givenchy, Marc Bohan, and Pierre Balmain all worked for him at one time or another. He closed his business down in 1951.

Parfums Robert Piguet was formed in 1942 and its first fragrance, Bandit, came out two years later, the first perfume to use a leathery base note. It was followed by three others, including, in 1948, Fracas, which contained a strong element of tuberose. Both Bandit and Fracas were created for Piguet by Roure's prominent woman "nose" Germaine Cellier, who formulated the classic Vent Vert for Balmain in 1945 and was also to create Jolie Madame for him later.

Like its creator, Fracas was a little eccentric, a little provocative, a little revolutionary, a little wild, but it was memorable. Fracas disappeared with the closure of the business and Piguet's death two years later. Only recently has the house and the perfume been revived The perfume is still contained in the opal black cube flacon, with a facetted crystal stopper, based on the original bottle.

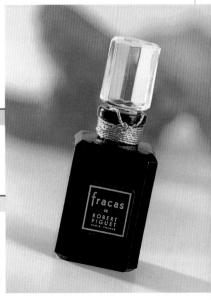

Fracas

LAUNCHED	*1948, relaunched 1998*
CREATOR	*Germaine Cellier*
CATEGORY	*floral fruity spicy*
FLACON	*n/a*

notes

TOP	*orange blossom, peach, bergamot, green notes*
MIDDLE	*tuberose, jasmine, iris, lily of the valley*
LOWER	*musk, cedar, sandalwood, oak moss, amber*

PARFUMS PACO RABANNE

Fragrances from a perfumer who is always keen to shock

PARENT COMPANY	*Antonio Puig*
HEADQUARTERS	*Paris, France*
CURRENT PERFUMES	*Calandre, XS pour Elle, Paco*

Paco Rabanne was born in 1934 in San Sebastian and was a refugee in France at the age of five. He studied architecture in Paris, but to earn money for this he designed fashion accessories such as purses and jewelry. In 1964 he presented a spectacular and revolutionary clothes collection to the Paris fashion world, with experimental dresses in contemporary materials such as metal and plastic. He went on to gain further notoriety with paper dresses, molded clothing, knitted fur, and clothes made of mirrors and laser discs.

He used models who danced in large-meshed chain-mail dresses with nothing underneath and the press could not resist him. Always keen to shock, he linked up with Antonio Puig in 1969 to produce what is now a classic perfume, Calandre—in French a car radiator grille. Using newly discovered chemicals, it introduced a subtle metal note into the accord and was presented in a bottle designed by Pierre Dinand which resembled a Rolls-Royce grille.

Other perfumes then followed: Métal in 1979; La Nuit in 1985; the award-winning linear fragrance XS pour Elle, in a bottle with a silver cap bearing astrological symbols; finally a unisex fragrance, Paco, which is sold without published detail in a plain aluminum can!

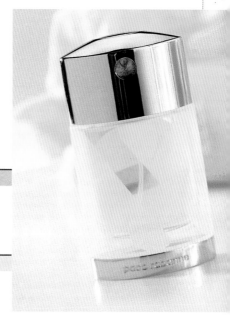

XS pour Elle

LAUNCHED	*1994*
CREATOR	*Firmenich*
CATEGORY	*floral*
FLACON	*Pierre Dinand*

notes

LINEAR	*water jasmine, freesia, peony, sandalwood, amber*

OSCAR DE LA RENTA

Award-winning creator of quality floral perfumes

PARENT COMPANY	*Sanofi (although company currently up for sale)*
HEADQUARTERS	*Paris, France*
CURRENT PERFUMES	*Oscar, Volupté, So de la Renta*

The very name Oscar de la Renta evokes the idea of sumptuous luxury and the most elegant sophistication. In origin he is an American-Dominican born in Santo Domingo in 1932, and he has an impeccable couture background.

After studying art in Madrid, he first worked for the Balenciaga and later the Lanvin couture houses, before establishing his own fashion house in New York in 1965, and in 1991 he was the first American designer to show his collections in Paris. In 1993 he was appointed head designer for Balmain.

He has twice been president of the Council of Fashion Designers of America, which in 1990 selected him for a Lifetime Achievement award. He has twice won the Coty American Fashion Critics award, and has

ABOVE: *The floral bouquet of So de la Renta.*

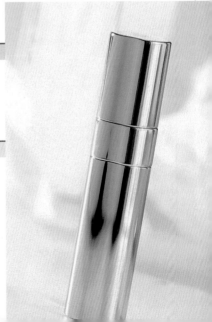

Oscar

LAUNCHED	*1977*
CREATOR	*Jean-Louis Sieuzac (Givaudan-Roure)*
CATEGORY	*floral oriental*
FLACON	*Pierre Dinand*

notes

TOP	*orange flower, basil, cilantro, cascarilla*
MIDDLE	*rose, tuberose, jasmine, ylang-ylang, broom*
LOWER	*opopanax, cloves, patchouli, sandalwood, vetiver, lavender, castoreum, myrrh*

So de la Renta

LAUNCHED *1997*

CREATOR *Ilias Ermenidis (Firmenich)*

CATEGORY *fruity spicy floral*

FLACON *Oscar de la Renta*

notes

TOP *cardamom, mango, kiwi, watermelon, clementine, freesia, gardenia*

MIDDLE *pimento leaves, sampaquita flower, narcissus, tuberose, peony, lotus*

LOWER *musk, plum, satinwood, vanilla*

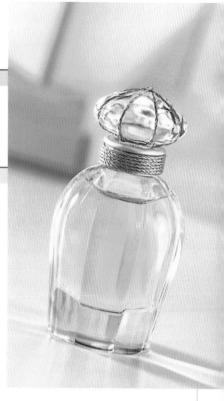

served on the boards of the Metropolitan Opera and of Carnegie Hall, in New York. From the base of his main boutique in the Rue du Faubourg in Paris, he is now behind a wide range of jewelry, purses, eyewear, swimwear, lingerie, millinery, umbrellas, and, of course, fragrances.

The fragrance side of Oscar de la Renta's business started in 1977, when he launched his signature perfume Oscar de la Renta, now called Oscar, which won two FiFi awards, including "best new women's fragrance," in the next year and a FiFi "perennial success" award in 1992. It was inspired by his childhood recollections of his mother's garden in Santo Domingo in days when he believed that a flower's dewdrops held the essence of its fragrance.

Volupté followed in 1992, another award-winning floral-oriental perfume, created this time by IFF perfumers, with strongly floral notes in the heart and a superb flacon, designed by Pierre Dinand, of very smooth, heavy glass ornamented with a gold band and an emerald stopper. Then, after a men's fragrance called Pour Lui, came So de la Renta, described as a "sheer luscious floral." These are all perfumes of superb quality. In 1995 Oscar de la Renta received the Living Legend award from the American Society of Perfumers.

NINA RICCI

Creator of a fragrance acclaimed as one of the five greatest perfumes in the world

PARENT COMPANY	*Antonio Puig*
HEADQUARTERS	*Paris, France*
CURRENT PERFUMES	*L'Air du Temps, Fleur de Fleurs, Nina, Deci Dela, Les Belles di Ricci*

This is one of the very big French perfume houses, but rather surprisingly Nina Ricci herself took no part in the perfume side of her business, nor indeed did she ever wear perfume. It was her son Robert who was the perfume man. Nina Ricci was born Marie Nielli (Nina being her childhood nickname) in Turin in 1883; she married a jeweler and opened the Paris couture house with Robert in 1932.

She continued designing elegant and extremely feminine dresses with great success until 1954 and she later died in 1970. Robert had taken over full control of the house after the war and decided to introduce fragrances to the business as an insurance against the uncertain economics of couture. It suited him very well because at heart he was already a perfumer, a romantic with a highly sensitive nose. The family also happened to be close friends of the Lalique family, who helped him to contain his scents in the most superb bottles. For a time, indeed, Lalique would make scent bottles only for Ricci.

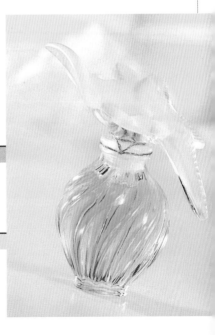

L'Air du Temps

LAUNCHED	*1948*
CREATOR	*Francis Fabron (Roure)*
CATEGORY	*floral*
FLACON	*Marc Lalique*

notes

TOP	*bergamot, carnation, rose*
MIDDLE	*gardenia, jasmine, rose, orris, ylang-ylang*
LOWER	*musk, iris, sandalwood*

Robert Ricci took a very firm hand in every aspect of the production of his perfumes, always knowing exactly what he wanted. He started with Coeur-Joie, which was launched in 1946 as a paean of triumph marking the end of the war and appeared in a heart-shaped flacon designed by Marc Lalique. Then, in 1948, came L'Air du Temps, which has been described as the perfect symbol of a fashion house whose name is synonymous with romanticism.

Together with Shalimar, Chanel No5, Arpège, and Joy, L'Air du Temps has been acclaimed as one of the five greatest perfumes in the world. There must be some truth in this, for it has been avowed too that one bottle of this fragrance was being sold somewhere in the world every second.

The creator of L'Air du Temps, Francis Fabron, who worked for the great fragrance manufacturing firm Roure-Bertrand-Dupont, now Givaudan Roure, was able to produce a fragrance that met Robert Ricci's requirements very early in what can sometimes be a very long process of selection, testing, and amendment. It was not a complex fragrance and its notes were clearly defined, using natural materials where possible. It was intended, as described by its creator, to leave a memory when the wearer passed by. The bottle was designed by Robert's close friend Marc Lalique and at first represented an oval sun in crystal, with a dove carved in relief on the stopper. The famous "dove bottle," with a pair of carved doves fluttering above the stopper, seen as a symbol of love and tenderness, was produced in 1951 but has had several variations.

In the following years Robert Ricci produced Capricci (1960), Mademoiselle Ricci (1967), Farouche (1973), Fleur de Fleurs (1980),

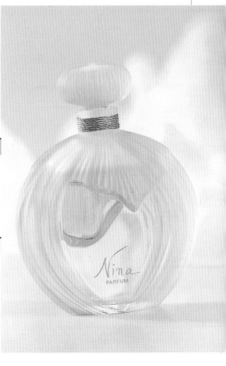

Nina

LAUNCHED	*1987*
CREATOR	*Christian Vacchiano (Argeville)*
CATEGORY	*floral*
FLACON	*Marie-Claude Lalique*

notes

TOP	*bergamot, mimosa, cassia tree buds, basil, orange blossom, marigold*
MIDDLE	*jasmine, mimosa, rose, violet, ylang-ylang*
LOWER	*iris, sandalwood, vetiver, cassis*

Deci Dela

LAUNCHED **1994**

CREATOR **Jean Guichard (Givaudan-Roure)**

CATEGORY **fruity floral chypre**

FLACON **Elizabeth Garouste and Mattia Bonetti**

notes

TOP **peach, raspberry, redcurrant, boronia, osmanthus**

MIDDLE **rose, sweet pea, freesia, hazelnut**

LOWER **sandalwood, patchouli, balsam, cypress, aloewood**

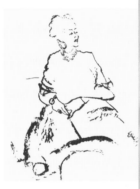

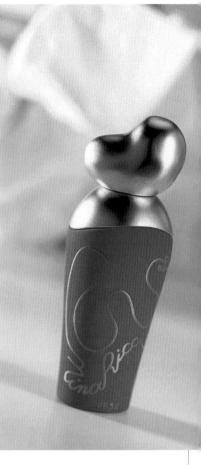

ABOVE: *Madame Nina Ricci.*

Nina (1987), Deci Dela (1995), and Les Belles de Ricci (1997). The fragrance, Nina, was Robert Ricci's tribute to his late mother and was an intentional reversion to the earlier traditions of perfumery in protest against the new, strong, modern fragrances like Giorgio Beverly Hills and Obsession, which he greatly disliked. It symbolized and was made for the more mature woman, aged perhaps 35 to 40, in contrast to the younger woman for whom he had made L'Air du Temps.

He had had the idea of Nina in mind for some while before a Grasse perfumer, who had been studying his likes and dislikes, presented him with a sample that perfectly matched his feelings. The bottle, representing folds of dress material, was designed by Marie-Claude Lalique. The perfume was a great success. Next year Robert Ricci died and Parfums Nina Ricci eventually passed to Sanofi and, in 1997, to the Spanish conglomerate Puig.

PARFUMS ROCHAS

The first perfume to be given the name of a living person

PARENT COMPANY	*Wella*
HEADQUARTERS	*Paris, France*
CURRENT PERFUMES	*Femme, Madame Rochas, Eau de Rochas, Mystère, Lumière, Byzance, Tocade, Byzantine, Fleur d'Eau, Toccadilly, Alchimie*

Marcel Rochas opened his own fashion house in Paris at the age of 22, encouraged by the great Art Deco designer of the time, Paul Parquet. It was 1925 and the frenetic days of the 1920s were moving into jazz, sports cars, and an emphasis on youth.

"My era was my guide," Rochas said about his style, and proceeded to slim down, tuck in, and replace wool with silk to create glamour. Soon his second home was Hollywood and his clients included Joan Crawford, Katherine Hepburn, and Marlene Dietrich.

Almost from the start Rochas had founded a perfume division alongside the couture business, launching several scents that have not lasted. But in 1944 he married a very beautiful girl, Hélène, and gave her, as a wedding present, a new perfume, the first creation of Edmond Roudnitska, now the doyen of the "noses." As soon as the end of the war permitted, Femme was launched for commercial sale, to

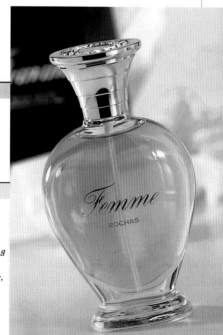

Femme

LAUNCHED	*1945*
CREATOR	*Edmond Roudnitska*
CATEGORY	*chypre*
FLACON	*Marcel Rochas and Lalique*

notes

TOP	*peach, plum, apricot, bergamot, cinnamon*
MIDDLE	*jasmine, rose, immortelle, ylang-ylang*
LOWER	*oak moss, sandalwood, patchouli, musk, amber, vanilla*

become an immediate success. The stylized female torso of the flacon is said to have been designed by Rochas himself and modeled on the curves of Mae West.

Marcel Rochas died in 1955 and his business partner decided to close down the fashion business but to keep the fragrance house going. In an inspired move he appointed Hélène Rochas president of the company. She was only 28. For some time she worked closely with another great perfumer, Guy Robert, to devise a fragrance for the woman of the 1960s. The graceful perfume called Madame Rochas was the result—a variation of the popular white-flowers theme, suited for both day and evening wear, with some 200 ingredients and an elegant container adapted by Pierre Dinand from an eighteenth-century smelling-salts bottle by Baccarat. The bottle was Dinand's first big commission and the perfume was the first to be given the name of a living person.

The company now appointed its own perfumer, Nicholas Mamounas, who was to create the Rochas fragrances for the next 20 years. Eau de Rochas, with sparkling notes of lime and verbena, appeared in 1970, then, in 1978, Mystère, a warm, haunting fragrance with floral and animalistic features drawn from some 200 ingredients. In 1984 the fresh, floral Lumière was launched, with green top notes and a heart containing gardenia, jasmine, and magnolia.

The last perfume created for Rochas by Nicholas Mamounas was Byzance, commemorating the Empire of Byzantium, the fusing of East and West

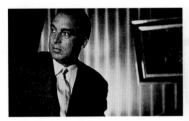

ABOVE: *Marcel Rochas.*

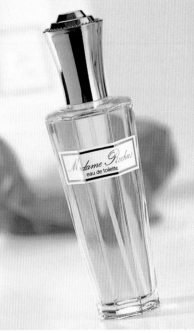

Madame Rochas

LAUNCHED *1960*
CREATOR *Guy Robert*
CATEGORY *floral aldehyde*
FLACON *Pierre Dinand / Rochas*

notes

TOP *orange blossom, broom, honeysuckle, neroli*
MIDDLE *ylang-ylang, tuberose, jasmine, orris, rose*
LOWER *sandalwood, cedar, musk, amber*

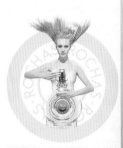

Alchimie

LAUNCHED *1998*

CREATOR *Jacques Cavallier (Firmenich)*

CATEGORY *described as "fresh floral-sensual"*

FLACON *Serge Mansau*

notes

TOP *lilac, cucumber, hyacinth, pear, mandarin, blackcurrant*

MIDDLE *coconut, wisteria, jasmine, tiaré, mallow, acacia*

LOWER *sandalwood, heliotrope, musk, amber, vanilla, tonka*

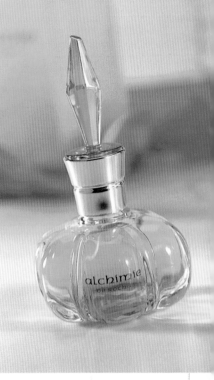

LEFT: *A notable advertisement for Byzantine.*

in a lush, rich combination, with a cobalt-blue bottle reflecting Byzantine mosaics and architecture. This theme was taken further with Byzantine in 1995, the bottle for this fragrance carried a laser-disc emblem symbolizing technology; these are intellectual perfumes!

When Rochas launched Tocade in 1994 their style was completely changed. Tocade, meaning "flirtation," was an innovative rose-vanilla-amber fragrance by Maurice Roucel (then with Quest) and Serge Mansau's bottle adapted the Femme flacon in a light-hearted manner with a collar and hat. Tocade has won five international fragrance awards. Toccadilly, in 1997, was specifically aimed at "the younger woman who is not afraid to enjoy life," focused as a seductive chessboard queen. It is presented in a bright Harlequin-colored bottle.

But the latest perfume, Alchimie, their last launch, Rochas claim, before the end of the century, reverts to a more romantic format stressing sensual passion; it was created by Jacques Cavallier, who made Poême for Lancôme.

ROYAL DOULTON

One of the best-known names in pottery, now the creator of a high-quality fragrance

PARENT COMPANY	**Brandselite International**
HEADQUARTERS	**Ontario, Canada**
CURRENT PERFUME	**Doulton**

Royal Doulton is one of the most prominent of Britain's long-established and highly distinguished pottery companies, with origins going back into the eighteenth century. It took on its present name a few years ago after an amalgamation of Doulton with two other older but similarly well-known companies, Minton and Royal Crown Derby. In their time all three companies have had interests in the perfume industry as the manufacturers of beautiful porcelain scent bottles for women's dressing tables.

Royal Crown Derby (founded around 1750) started to produce these in the late eighteenth century; Minton (founded in 1796) was making bottles with flower-encrusted decoration by 1830; and Doulton, the newest of the three companies, started to make bottles of salt-glazed stoneware, decorated with sunflowers and foliage, in 1900.

Now Royal Doulton has gone a further stage and brought out a high-quality perfume called Doulton, which is produced by a Canadian licensee in Ontario in a beautiful spherical flacon for the Royal Doulton Fine Fragrance Collection.

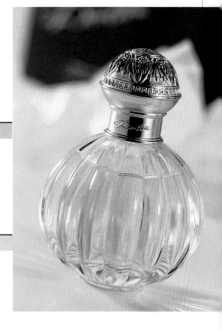

Doulton

LAUNCHED *1998*
CREATOR *Patricia Bilodeau (Dragoco)*
CATEGORY *floriental*
FLACON *Shikatani Lacroix Design, Toronto*

notes

TOP *melon, plum*
MIDDLE *muguet, narcissus, lily*
LOWER *sandalwood, amber, musk, patchouli*

PARFUMS YVES SAINT LAURENT

Called the "greatest fashion designer in the world" and creator of controversial fragrances

PARENT COMPANY	*Sanofi*
HEADQUARTERS	*Paris, France*
CURRENT PERFUMES	*Y, Rive Gauche, Opium, Paris, Yvresse, In Love Again, Vice Versa*

Since its foundation, Yves Saint Laurent has launched five fragrances for women; all have been notable but two have presented the company with considerable problems. Saint Laurent was born in Algeria in 1936 and started making clothes, for his sister's dolls, at the age of seven.

He attended an *haute couture* training college in Paris and, at the age of 18, won both first and third prizes in an International Wool Secretariat design competition. His talent was recognized by Michel Brünhoff, a director of *Vogue*, who introduced him to Christian Dior. Dior had never had a design assistant before, but immediately took on Yves Saint Laurent as the head of his design team. Yves later admitted that Dior was "a prodigious master who taught him the roots of his art."

When Dior died suddenly in 1957, Yves Saint Laurent became artistic director, producing successful collections until 1960, when an attempt to draw the street scene into fashion was a disaster. The young designer was then called up for a period of military service.

In 1962 Saint Laurent returned to form his own house with a business partner, Pierre Bergé, and financial support from an Atlanta businessman who took 80 percent

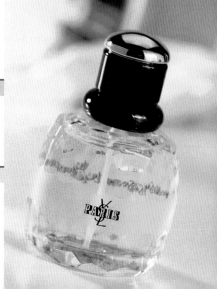

Paris

LAUNCHED	*1983*
CREATOR	*Sophia Grosjman (IFF)*
CATEGORY	*floral*
FLACON	*Alain de Morgues*

notes

TOP	*mimosa, geranium, hawthorn, cassie*
MIDDLE	*rose, violet, orris*
LOWER	*sandalwood, amber, musk*

Opium

LAUNCHED	*1977*
CREATORS	*Jean Amic and Jean-Louis Sieuzac (Roure)*
CATEGORY	*oriental*
FLACON	*Pierre Dinand*

notes

TOP	*mandarin, plum, clove, pepper, cilantro*
MIDDLE	*lily of the valley, rose, jasmine*
LOWER	*labdanum, benzoin, myrrh, opopanax, castoreum, cedar, sandalwood*

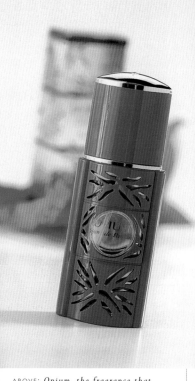

ABOVE: *Opium, the fragrance that knocked tradition.*

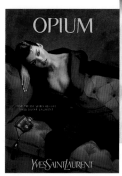

of the shares. His fashion collections were successful and by 1971 he was being called "the greatest fashion designer in the world." His company now has stores worldwide and fame has extended to his work on costumes and settings in films and the theater.

Saint Laurent's first perfume was Y (the continental *Ee-grek*). Created by Jean Amic of Roure and in a bottle by Pierre Dinand, this was an innovative style of chypre perfume, introduced in 1964. Rive Gauche, an aldehydic floral also created by Roure perfumers, followed in 1971. After a visit to the Far East, Saint Laurent decided to produce a perfume reminiscent of Imperial China—oriental, mysterious, and heavy—which he would call Opium. To him that name evoked the right Oriental setting rather than the drug. Unfortunately his American financier had sold his majority shareholding in the company to Charles of the Ritz, itself owned by the mighty and very conservative Squibb Corporation. Squibb were horrified by the implications of this name and protested; Saint Laurent insisted, but it was a long time before he won his argument. Fears of continued protest in the USA led to a decision to delay the

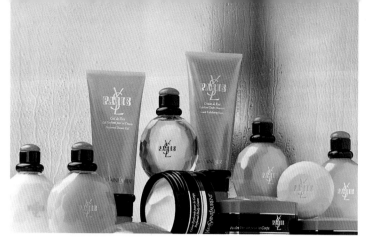

ABOVE: *Variety of products in the Paris bath line.*

launch in America for a year after that in Europe, where it was was a huge success. Finally introduced into the US, with an ultra lavish party on the sailing ship *Peking*, it was again extraordinarily successful and has been Yves Saint Laurent's best-selling perfume ever since.

Yves got his revenge. In 1986 he managed to buy Charles of the Ritz back, retained Parfums Yves Saint Laurent, and sold the rest of the business on to Revlon. His company is now part of the Sanofi group but they have recently put the company up for sale.

Paris, the next Saint Laurent perfume, came out with a flourish in 1983 and set a trend, this time a return to romance and femininity, with the fragrance of roses. The exact rose effect Yves Saint Laurent wanted was hard to capture and there were many trials before a young perfumer in IFF came up with the right answer. Her name was Sophia Grosjman, now one of the foremost perfumers in the world. It was her first creation. Champagne followed. The selection of this name was vigorously opposed by the winemakers. After long and hard-fought court proceedings, the name, and to an extent the bottle design, had to be changed. It is now called Yvresse.

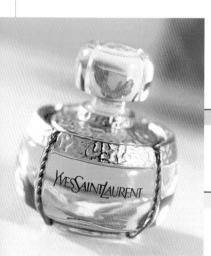

Yvresse

LAUNCHED	*1993*
CREATOR	*Sophia Grosjman (IFF)*
CATEGORY	*fruity floral chypre*
FLACON	*Joël Desgrippes*

notes

TOP	*nectarine, mint, anise*
MIDDLE	*rose, litchi*
LOWER	*patchouli, vetiver, oak moss*

JIL SANDER

The designer who went on to produce a women's perfume with masculine notes

PARENT COMPANY	*Lancaster / Coty*
HEADQUARTERS	*Paris, France*
CURRENT PERFUMES	*Woman III, Woman No. 4, Jil*

Jil Sander is a German designer who studied textile design in Hamburg, worked in Los Angeles as a journalist, became a fashion editor in Germany in 1968, and, at the age of 25, started to design clothes. She sold her car to buy her first store, which was just round the corner from where her large corporate headquarters building now stands.

Jil Sander entered the fragrance market in 1980 when she launched a signature fragrance, Jil Sander. She followed this in 1983 with Woman Two, then Woman III, which has been described as a woman's perfume with masculine notes (for example oak moss, cedar, tonka, and musk), in 1987, and Woman No. 4, a floriental with fruity scents, in 1991. The two latter fragrances were composed for her by perfumers of Créations Aromatiques in bottles designed by Peter Schmidt. In 1997 she launched a new signature perfume, called simply Jil.

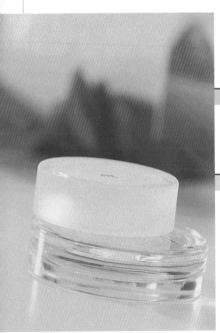

Jil

LAUNCHED	*1997*
CREATOR	*Gilles Romey (Quest)*
CATEGORY	*oriental aromatic*
FLACON	*Fabien Baron*

notes

TOP	*lavender, violet, raspberry*
MIDDLE	*cedar, vetiver, fir, sandalwood*
LOWER	*ambergris, vanilla*

SCHIAPARELLI

Creator of a shocking fragrance, reflecting her trademarks of panache and eccentricity

PARENT COMPANY	*Parfums de Marque*
HEADQUARTERS	*Paris, France*
CURRENT PERFUMES	*Shocking, Zut, Lancetti*

The immediate thought of most people when asked about Elsa Schiaparelli is a color, "shocking pink." She was born in Rome in 1890, married a French count, went to Paris, fell in with the Dada movement, and entered the world of fashion by creating a range of knitwear in startling new colors. Her sweaters, cardigans, and skirts attracted enthusiastic attention and sold rapidly, especially in the USA.

She opened her own couture house in 1928 and for many years it was a center for those in the *avant-garde* of art and fashion in Paris. Color, panache, eccentricity, and surrealism were her trademarks.

Schiaparelli had produced two perfumes in her earlier years, but Shocking, made to accompany her "shocking-pink" clothes collection, proved a sensation. It was a voluptous scent, but, as with all her

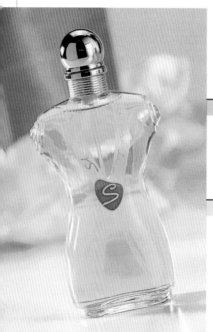

Shocking

LAUNCHED	*1937 and 1998*
CREATOR	*Jean Carles (1998 by Dragoco perfumers)*
CATEGORY	*oriental*
FLACON	*after the original*

notes

TOP	*hyacinth, ylang-ylang, narcissus*
MIDDLE	*rose, jasmine, lily of the valley*
LOWER	*sandalwood, patchouli, amber, musk*

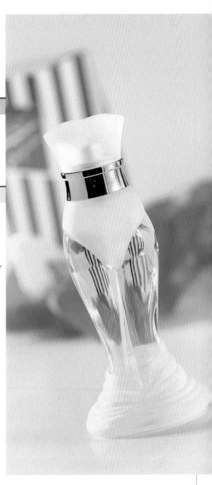

Zut

LAUNCHED *1949 and 1998*
CREATOR *now Givaudan-Roure*
CATEGORY *green fruity floral*
FLACON *after the original*

notes

TOP *ylang-ylang,*
blackcurrant, linden
MIDDLE *jasmine, lily of the*
valley, rose, iris, incense
LOWER *vanilla, musk, and woody*
notes

fragrances, it was really the bottle that drew attention. The Shocking flacon was a model of a corseted female torso derived from the tailor's dummy she had made for Mae West. Other perfumes followed with equally surprising containers: Sleeping, for example, in a Baccarat bottle shaped like a candle, and Roy Soleil in a famous "blazing sun" bottle designed for her by Salvador Dali to celebrate the end of World War II. Schiaparelli's reaction to Dior's New Look fashion was the laconic, "Et puis, Zut," which she expressed in a scent with a bottle showing the lower half of the Shocking torso, allegedly with the legs of Mistinguette (a French actress and dancer, 1875–1956). There were others.

Elsa Schiaparelli died in 1973 and, although her perfume company produced one or two more fragrances, business slumped. The company, associated with Pikenz, is now in the hands of new owners who are reviving some of her great early successes, starting with Shocking and Zut. Both are being sold at *eau de parfum* concentration in bottles derived from the originals.

SHISEIDO

The world's largest cosmetics company, which integrates science with art in its products

PARENT COMPANY	*independent*
HEADQUARTERS	*Tokyo, Japan*
CURRENT PERFUMES	*Feminité du Bois, Relaxing Fragrance, Vocalise, Musc Koublaï Khän, Rähat Loukoum*

As a pharmacy, Shiseido goes a long way back into history, for it was founded in Tokyo by Yushin Fukuhara in 1872. But it did not start making perfume until after World War II and its first sales of fragrances overseas, to the United States, did not begin until the early 1960s. Another 20 years then passed before it put a commercial foot inside Europe.

Shiseido is now the world's largest cosmetics company and it also owns two distinguished perfume houses which are run separately, Issey Miyake and Jean-Paul Gaultier. Shiseido's European subsidiary, Beauté Prestige International, is based at Bolougne-Billancourt in France, and it has exclusive stores in Les Salons du Palais Royal in Paris and elsewhere.

The Shiseido company has always attached importance to the integration of science with art in its products, and in 1960 founded the Shiseido Design Department, at present directed by the artist Serge Lutens. Some of the Shiseido advertisements over recent years have been outstanding.

Feminité du Bois

LAUNCHED	*1992*
CREATOR	*Pierre Bourdon and Christopher Sheldrake (Quest)*
CATEGORY	*leathery, woody*
FLACON	*Serge Lutens*

notes

TOP	*orange blossom, rose, cedarwood*
MIDDLE	*peach, honey, beeswax, violet, cedarwood*
LOWER	*cardamom, cinnamon, clove, musk, vanilla, cedarwood*

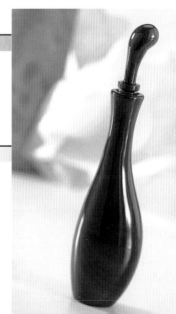

Vocalise

LAUNCHED *1998*

CREATOR *Jacques Cavallier (Firmenich)*

CATEGORY *fresh floral oriental*

FLACON *Aoshi Kudo*

notes

LINEAR *orchid, vanilla, cassis, yuzu lemon, pepper, rose, neroli, muguet, peach, musk, hinoki*

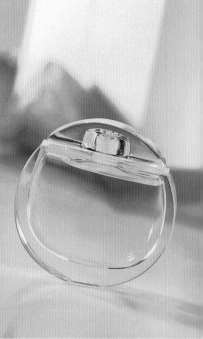

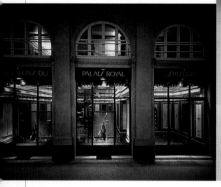

ABOVE: *Shisheido's store in Les Salons du Palais Royal, Paris.*

Shiseido have also been pioneers in aromachology, the study of the physical aspects and effects of fragrances and especially their calming or uplifting qualities. An aromatic alarm clock, which emits a pleasant smell to wake you up in a good mood, is one example. The emission of fragrances in a factory or office to relieve stress on workers is another. The perfume Relaxing is a direct outcome of this interest.

Although a number of fragrances were sold when Shiseido first tested their products on the European market, and a few had previously been sold in the USA as well, Shiseido's first real attempt to sell outside their established market in the Far East came with Feminité du Bois in 1992. This scent, described as a "pure, sensual fragrance inspired by the strength of women," has a cedarwood note running throughout, is designed for all occasions, and claims to promote a general sense of wellbeing. In 1997 the company launched Relaxing Fragrance (also just called Relaxing), this stressed the aromachology aspect of scent, with notes designed to provide "a world of relaxation and renewal," especially from spices and a strong sandalwood base note. Vocalise followed in 1998, composed in a new format by which the notes are said to develop around a core fragrance of oriental style.

ALFRED SUNG

Creators of Forever, a rhapsody of florals and a harmony of contrasts

PARENT COMPANY	*Riviera Concepts*
HEADQUARTERS	*Ontario, Canada, and New York, USA*
CURRENT PERFUMES	*Sung, Sung Forever, Sung Pure*

In 1989 the classical fashion designer Alfred Sung launched a signature fragrance of high quality in the floral-green family. Sung came out at the same time as Ralph Lauren's Safari, a perfume in the same category, but the marketing skills and finance behind the latter overwhelmed Alfred Sung's little product, so that the one was soon famous whereas the other sold principally to "those in the know" and for a time ceased to be sold in the UK at all.

However, it was in due course acquired by a Canadian perfume company, Riviera Concepts, which has now brought about the revival of the Alfred Sung perfume house by adding two new perfumes, Forever in 1995 and Pure in 1997.

Sung has a citrusy head on a floral heart with musk and woody notes to provide the depth. Pure, a woody floral, uses tangerine and orchid above a white floral bouquet, with a warm ambery base. Forever is described as a rhapsody of florals and a harmony of contrasts, appearing in a classically simple bottle, made at up to *parfum* concentration.

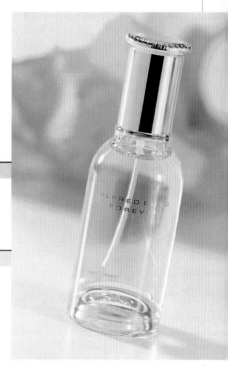

Sung Forever

LAUNCHED	*1995*
CREATOR	*Dragoco perfumers*
CATEGORY	*floral*
FLACON	*Pierre Dinand*

notes

TOP	*plum, tayberry, peony buds*
MIDDLE	*freesia, narcissus, rose, lily of the valley*
LOWER	*mahonia, sandalwood, amber*

ELIZABETH TAYLOR

Two award-winning fragrances, each with a success story to tell . . .

PARENT COMPANY	*Parfums International / Elizabeth Arden*
HEADQUARTERS	*New York, USA*
CURRENT PERFUMES	*White Diamonds, Black Pearls*

It must always have seemed a safe bet that if a perfume were to be issued carrying the name of a megastar like Elizabeth Taylor a lot of people would buy it. The point was proved in 1988, when Elizabeth Taylor's Passion won a FiFi award for the most successful women's fragrance. It was proved again in 1992, when the second fragrance carrying her name, Elizabeth Taylor's White Diamonds, was put on the market and promptly won two FiFi awards (for Best Woman's Fragrance Introduction and Best TV Advertising Campaign). White Diamonds has been one of the great success stories, exceeding all market expectations; in Selfridges, in London, for example, it was the 1992 best-selling fragrance, a success repeated all over the world. It has been one of the top-selling quality perfumes ever since in the United States.

Parfums International have issued a number of other Elizabeth Taylor perfumes since, which have now been discontinued, but Black Pearls, based on an accord of peach and gardenia and launched in 1996, is sold in the USA though no longer in the UK.

White Diamonds

LAUNCHED	*1992*
CREATOR	*Sophia Grosjman (IFF)*
CATEGORY	*floral*
FLACON	*Susan Wacker (Parfums International)*

notes

TOP	*lily, neroli, aldehydes*
MIDDLE	*tuberose, narcissus, rose, jasmine, orris*
LOWER	*amber, oak moss, patchouli, sandalwood*

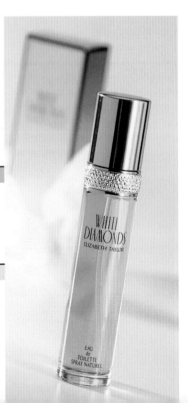

TIFFANY & CO.

An award-winning perfume from the house that caters to the cream of American society

PARENT COMPANY	*independent*
HEADQUARTERS	*New York, USA*
CURRENT PERFUMES	*Tiffany, Trueste*

When Charles Lewis Tiffany opened his New York store in 1837 he sold umbrellas, pottery, and Chinese bric-a-brac. But he was a man with flair and great ideas. By 1854, when the great American silversmith John Moore became a partner, his business was set to become one of the most famous jewelers and silversmiths in the world, offering customers exquisite gold, silver, and diamond jewelry, together with watches, silverware, and the famous Tiffany clocks, all made to an exceptionally high standard. Tiffany customers include everybody who is anybody in American society.

In 1987, to celebrate its 150th birthday, the company launched a women's fragrance called Tiffany, which was made up to *parfum* concentration and appeared in a dramatic crystal flacon with gold and metallic inlays echoing the Art Deco façade of Tiffany's New York store. The success of this fragrance, which won FiFi awards in 1988 for both the perfume and the bottle, led to Trueste, launched in 1995, a fruity-floral perfume in a bottle incorporating a Tiffany "jewel" cap and gold collar.

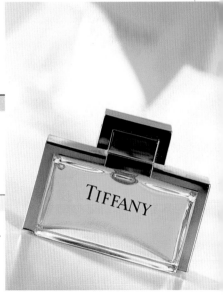

Tiffany

LAUNCHED	*1987*
CREATOR	*François Demachy (Chanel)*
CATEGORY	*fruity floral*
FLACON	*Pierre Dinand*

notes

TOP	*mandarin, cassis*
MIDDLE	*rose, jasmine, iris, ylang-ylang, orange blossom, muguet, violet leaves*
LOWER	*sandalwood, vetiver, amber, vanilla*

PARFUMS TRUSSARDI

The perfume house whose fragrances come in simple but elegant bottles

PARENT COMPANY	*International Cosmetics and Parfum*
HEADQUARTERS	*Milan, Italy*
CURRENT PERFUMES	*Trussardi, Trussardi Action (in Italy only), Donna Trussardi, Trussardi Light Her*

The empire of Nicola Trussardi started in Milan before World War I, when his grandfather opened a business designing leather gloves. Nicola himself, born in 1942, is now a designer on the grand scale, designing everything from fashion clothing to telephones, from suitcases to store and aircraft interiors. Most of his products carry a personal trademark, a little greyhound head mascot. His worldwide interests now include over 150 Trussardi stores.

Trussardi entered the fragrance market in the late 1970s, founding Parfums Trussardi and launching his signature perfume, Trussardi, also now known as Trussardi Classic, in 1980. Trussardi Action came in 1990, with a unisex variant of that in 1995, and the well-known Donna Trussardi, a floral chypre created by Jean Guichard of Givaudan-Roure, was launched in 1994.

The latest is Trussardi Light (with a male version), intended as a celebration of youth. All Trussardi fragrances come in simple but elegant bottles by the prominent Italian glassmaker Bormioli Rocco.

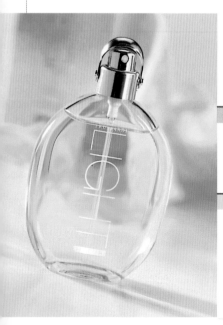

Trussardi Light Her

LAUNCHED	*1997*
CREATOR	*IFF perfumers*
CATEGORY	*floral fruity woody*
FLACON	*Bormioli Rocco*

notes

TOP	*yuzu lemon, lime, nectarine, quince flower*
MIDDLE	*freesia, lotus, waterlily, cyclamen, wisteria, peony, rose*
LOWER	*berries, apricot, sandalwood, patchouli, iris*

PARFUMS UNGARO

The house whose link with Chanel ensures perfumes of the highest quality

PARENT COMPANY	*Parfums Bvlgari*
HEADQUARTERS	*Geneva, Switzerland*
CURRENT PERFUMES	*Diva, Fleur de Diva*

Emmanuel Ungaro opened a couture house in Paris in 1965, launched his signature fragrance, the floral-woody Ungaro, in 1977, and in 1983 formed the perfume house Parfums Ungaro, which was subsequently acquired from him by Chanel. The link with Chanel meant that all of Chanel's perfume facilities could be utilized, including the services of their two prominent perfumers, Jacques Polge and François Demachy. As a result, Ungaro perfumes have always been of the highest quality.

Diva was launched in 1984 and became a considerable success, not least because of its attractive bottle, designed to suggest the folds of a woman's dress. A floral-spicy-amber scent called Senso came out in 1987 and three years later Ungaro was reformulated, with an alternative name Ungaro d'Ungaro, in a bottle designed by Jacques Helleu. There were male counterparts to these scents and also a unisex fragrance, Ombre de la Nuit. But, at the time of writing, the Ungaro position is uncertain, because the perfume house was acquired by Ferregamo (see page 91) in 1996 and has been linked up with Bvlgari. The full effects of this remain to be seen.

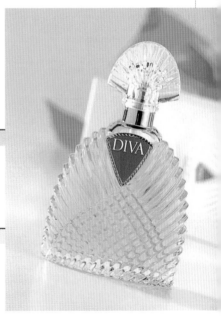

Diva

LAUNCHED	*1984*
CREATOR	*Jacques Polge*
CATEGORY	*floral amber*
FLACON	*Emmanuel Ungaro with Jacques Helleu*

notes

TOP	*tuberose, cardamom, mandarin, ylang-ylang*
MIDDLE	*orris, narcissus, jasmine*
LOWER	*sandalwood, patchouli, oak moss*

PARFUMS VALENTINO

Elegant fragrances from the couturier whose sophistication gives women style

PARENT COMPANY	*Parfums International / Elizabeth Arden*
HEADQUARTERS	*New York, USA*
CURRENT PERFUMES	*Classic Valentino, Vendetta pour Femme, Very Valentino*

Very Valentino

LAUNCHED	*1997*
CREATOR	*Daniella Roche (Givaudan Roure)*
CATEGORY	*hesperidic floral*
FLACON	*Pierre Dinand*

notes

TOP	*citrus, magnolia, lily of the valley*
MIDDLE	*jasmine, rose, woody notes*
LOWER	*sandalwood, vanilla, musk, amber*

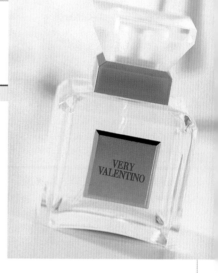

The famous Italian couturier Valentino Garavani was born in 1933 and has been prominent in the world of fashion and *haute couture* since the early 1960s. His customers are the jet set, film stars, and women of high society, the glamourous and the rich, for whom he creates sophisticated and exclusive gowns on top of the dresses of high quality and elegance sold from his stores in the major capitals. He has clothed Jackie Onassis, Elizabeth Taylor, Joan Collins, Sophia Loren, and Queen Noor of Jordan. He is a man who gives women style.

In 1977, through his perfume company Parfums Valentino, he introduced his signature perfume, Valentino, which is now called Classic Valentino. Vendetta, a very rich floral perfume created by IFF perfumers and marketed in a bottle made to resemble a fan pleat, was launched in 1993. In 1997 Very Valentino was put on the market, an essentially floral *eau de toilette* targeted at women aged 25–45 and aiming at "modern elegance with a hint of provocation." It comes in a flacon of cut crystal appearance.

VAN CLEEF & ARPELS

World-famous jewelers—creators of several distinguished fragrances

PARENT COMPANY	*Sanofi (although the company is now up for sale)*
HEADQUARTERS	*Paris, France*
CURRENT PERFUMES	*First, Van Cleef, Gem, Miss Arpels*

The House of Van Cleef & Arpels was set up in the Place Vendôme in Paris in 1906 to sell jewelry, which is still its main business. On its way to becoming a jewelry house of great prestige, it invented a revolutionary technique for eliminating any signs of metal used to mount precious stones and in 1949 it created a unique and extremely successful wristwatch.

It set up a store in New York in 1938 and thereafter began to expand all over the world. Van Cleef & Arpels went into the perfume market in 1976 with the opening of Parfums Van Cleef & Arpels and the launch of a distinguished floral-aldehydic perfume called First, created by a leading perfumer, Jean-Claude Ellena of Givaudan, and issued in a most elegant bottle designed by Jacques Llorente.

Their next venture, Gem, brought out in 1987, is a floral-oriental of fine quality, while their third, Van Cleef, inspired by the diamond and also a floral-oriental, has a multifaceted diamond-shaped bottle. The latest perfume from this house is Miss Arpels, a fruity-floral inspired by "a breath of fresh air in a florist's shop."

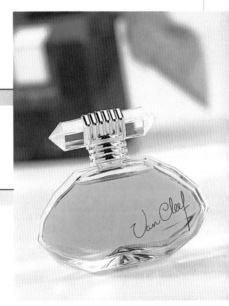

Van Cleef

LAUNCHED	*1994*
CREATOR	*Pascal Giraux (Haarmann & Reimer)*
CATEGORY	*floral oriental*
FLACON	*Serge Mansau*

notes

TOP	*bergamot, raspberry, neroli, tagette*
MIDDLE	*rose, jasmine, orange blossom, geranium*
LOWER	*cedar, tonka, vanilla, sandalwood*

VERSACE PROFUMI

The fragrance in a diamond—one of several perfumes in startlingly original bottles

PARENT COMPANY	*independent*
HEADQUARTERS	*Milan, Italy*
CURRENT PERFUMES	*Gianni Versace, V'E, Versus Donna, Blonde, three perfumes in Versace Jeans series, V/S*

Gianni Versace was born in southern Italy and when he was shot dead in Miami in 1997 he was only 50 years old. He was often seen as a rival to Giorgio Armani, who was 12 years his senior, but would dismiss that comparison with the following statement, "He is north. I am south. There is nothing to discuss."

From his youth he felt an affinity with the ancient Greek relics in his boyhood Calabria, symbolized by the Medusa head and Greek key-pattern surround used as his emblem and reflected in many of his designs. He learned dressmaking from his mother and started work as a designer in Milan, showing his first own-name collection in 1978.

By the end of the 1980s his bright, flamboyant, Baroque style could be recognized everywhere and he was designing costumes for opera and ballet as well as for fashion. He was always close to his sister, the striking-looking Donatella, whom he described as his muse, and it was no surprise when she carried on with his business interests seamlessly after his death.

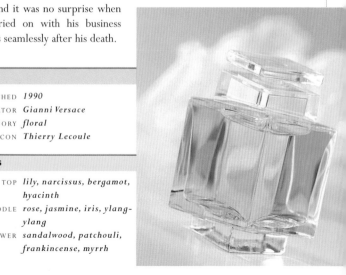

V'E

LAUNCHED	*1990*
CREATOR	*Gianni Versace*
CATEGORY	*floral*
FLACON	*Thierry Lecoule*

notes

TOP	*lily, narcissus, bergamot, hyacinth*
MIDDLE	*rose, jasmine, iris, ylang-ylang*
LOWER	*sandalwood, patchouli, frankincense, myrrh*

Blonde

LAUNCHED *1996*

CREATORS *Givaudan-Roure perfumers*

CATEGORY *floral*

FLACON *Serge Mansau*

notes

LINEAR *tuberose, violet, neroli, daffodil, violet leaves, orange flower, iris, broom, everlasting flower*

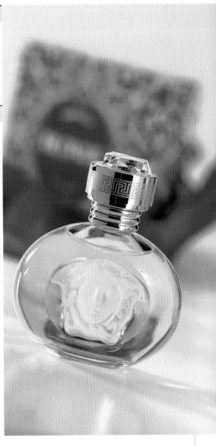

He clothed Madonna, Bianca Jagger, Lisa Marie Presley, and Linda Evangelista. His circle included Maurice Béjart and Elton John and he had lavish homes in Miami, Como, Milan, and New York. In the latter years of his life he designed towels and bedclothes, table linen and cushions, rugs, lamps, jewels, dinner services, and glassware. He wrote books, produced "that dress" for Elizabeth Hurley and was said to be able to predict today the fashion for the day after tomorrow.

Fragrance had been a part of Gianni Versace's business life from an early stage, his first perfume for women, called Gianni Versace, being launched in 1981, and considerable attention was always paid to the flacon designs. Gianni Versace, a floral-chypre, came in a notable diamond-shaped bottle with 56 facets on a prism-shaped base. In 1989 he introduced the perfume V'E in a highly original and elaborate "tilted cube" flacon designed by the young perfume-bottle designer Thierry Lecoule and made in a limited edition by Baccarat. Versus Donna, a powdery-fruity floral, was launched in 1993 in a bright scarlet bottle. Blonde, dedicated to his sister Donatella, reproduced the Medusa head on the side with the Greek key design on the cap. From 1994 onward he introduced a series of fragrances, half for young men and half for young women, called Versace Jeans, which were made to complement his Jeans label for young people and appeared in apparent soft-drink bottles inside tin cans. V/S was launched in the US at the end of 1998. The perfume house was Versace Profumi.

MADELEINE VIONNET

*Named for an extraordinary employer, in a bottle featuring thimbles
and fabric*

PARENT COMPANY	*independent*
HEADQUARTERS	*Paris, France*
CURRENT PERFUME	*Madeleine Vionnet*

This is a rare instance of a perfume issued in memory of an eminent designer who has long been dead. Madeleine Vionnet was born in 1876 and died in 1975. She opened the fashion house of Vionnet in Paris, France, in 1912 and by the early 1920s had 1,000 employees in 20 workshops.

She was a brilliant, innovative, *avant-garde* designer, the first to free women from corsets, the first to use the bias cut. She kept 15 models permanently showing her collections to clients. She was also a remarkable employer for her time, introducing unheard-of benefits like coffee breaks and paid holidays, even a dentist's surgery and an infirmary, for her staff.

Christian Dior admitted that "the art of couture was never taken further or higher" than by Vionnet, while Karl Lagerfeld has observed, "Everybody, whether he wants to be or not, is influenced by her." Her business closed in 1939.

In 1925 Vionnet introduced her first perfume, Temptation; others were simply named A, B, C, and D. The new perfume from Parfums Madeleine Vionnet follows the lines of Temptation, with a fascinating bottle featuring thimbles and fabric.

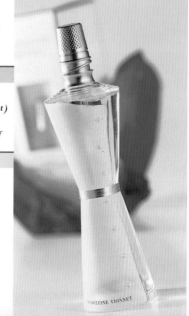

Madeleine Vionnet

LAUNCHED *1997*
CREATOR *Françoise Caron (Quest)*
CATEGORY *floral*
FLACON *Thierry de Bashmakoff*

notes

TOP *rose*
MIDDLE *peach flower,
osmanthus, tuberose,
rose, ylang-ylang*
LOWER *amber, myrrh, cedar,
sandalwood, musk*

VIVIENNE WESTWOOD

The designer who created a sensual fragrance to "transform the woman who wore it"

PARENT COMPANY	*Lancaster/Coty*
HEADQUARTERS	*London, England*
CURRENT PERFUME	*Boudoir*

The prominent London fashion designer Vivienne Westward, who started business in King's Road, Chelsea, even before punk and showed her first Paris collection in the early 1980s, has become a legend in her own lifetime, but she really belongs to a combination of tomorrow with the seventeenth and eighteenth centuries.

It is these early days that most emerge in her perfume Boudoir, launched in 1998. She has admitted that she wanted it to "transform the woman who wore it with the realization of her own sensuality" and to "reproduce everyone's idea of sex" and the French boudoir background found in the paintings of artists like Boucher suited this very well.

The opening notes use the scent of viburnum, extracted here for the first time by head space technology, and a striking flacon takes the shape of a glass pedestal supporting a regal orb, Vivienne Westwood's symbol, which is surmounted with a gold and jeweled Maltese cross and a Saturn-like ring. The perfume is made in both *parfum* and *eau de parfum* concentrations.

Boudoir

LAUNCHED	*1998*
CREATOR	*Martin Gras (Dragoco)*
CATEGORY	*floral oriental*
FLACON	*Fabrice Legros*

notes

TOP	*viburnum, French marigold*
MIDDLE	*rose, orris, orange blossom, cardamom, cilantro*
LOWER	*sandalwood, patchouli, vanilla, tobacco flower*

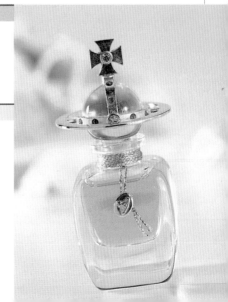

LES PARFUMS WORTH

Sensuous fragrances from the house founded by the father of haute couture

PARENT COMPANY	*International Classic Brands*
HEADQUARTERS	*London, England, and Paris, France*
CURRENT PERFUMES	*Je Reviens, Sans Adieu, Miss Worth*

At the age of 19 Charles Worth, a draper from Lincolnshire, England, went to Paris and took a job in a dress store, where he fell in love with another sales assistant, Marie Vernet. The dresses he designed for Marie to wear in the store attracted much attention—so much, indeed, that he decided to open his own couture house. He is now generally regarded as the father of *haute couture*.

Worth had married Marie and just before he died, in 1895, his two sons, Gaston and Jean-Philippe, took over the running of the house. In 1922 Jean-Philippe's son Jacques decided to supplement dresses with perfume. He was lucky enough to have two invaluable friends who joined him in the project—Maurice Blanchet, the perfumer, and René Lalique, the glassmaker.

Two years were spent developing a fragrance to evoke the sensuous feeling of nights on the Riviera and in 1925 they launched Dans la Nuit, in a ball-shaped, rich blue Lalique bottle, quickly followed by Vers le Jour. A wonderful sequence of other scents by Maurice Blanchet followed, including Sans Adieu and Je Reviens, almost all in Lalique flacons. Dans la Nuit was relaunched in 1985. The company now belongs to David Reiner but has recently been put up for sale.

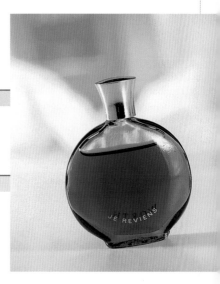

Je Reviens

LAUNCHED	*1932*
CREATOR	*Maurice Blanchet*
CATEGORY	*floral aldehyde*
FLACON	*Lalique*

notes

TOP	*jasmine, orange blossom, ylang-ylang, aldehydes*
MIDDLE	*narcissus, jonquil*
LOWER	*violet, sandalwood, vetiver, musk*

GLOSSARY

Absolute The essential oil of scented flowers and other aromatic plant parts in its very purest and most concentrated form. It is extremely expensive. See *Concrete*

Accord A combination of scents that blend together to produce a new fragrance (as when blue and yellow make green in painting).

Aldehyde An important group of very strong chemicals, mostly derived from alcohol, which are used in composing modern perfumes. They help to reproduce the odors of certain plants, provide individual scents of their own, and will enrich and strengthen a fragrance. Aldehyde chemicals were first used in Chanel No5.

Amber A fragrance found in ambergris and in other natural materials such as labdanum (not the fossilized resin used in jewelry). See *Oriental*

Aromachology The study of the effects of scents on people (for example, to calm or uplift them).

Aromatherapy The therapeutic treatment of people by applying essential oils from aromatic plants by massage or inhalation.

Aromatic In general, a plant or fragrance with a spicy note. More specifically in perfumery it describes the fragrance of certain herbs such as lavender or rosemary mainly used when producing men's fragrances. It can also simply mean "exuding a scent."

Atomizer A spray or vaporizer (some are now collectors' pieces).

Attar Also called otto. Essential oil obtained from a flower, in particular from the rose, by distillation.

Balsam Also called balm. A thick, viscous, gumlike exudation from certain plants which is used in perfumes for its sweet honey-like fragrance (for example, Balsam of tolu).

Bdellium An aromatic gum obtained from certain tropical trees (such as opopanax).

Bouquet A mixture of floral notes in a perfume. Also a perfume made from a mixture of perfume families.

Chypre The name of an important perfume made in Cyprus from Roman times and in Italy from the Middle Ages. Nowadays it designates one of the main perfume families, in which top notes (such as bergamot) and a floral heart (such as rose) are added to a woody, ambery base (for instance, oak moss, patchouli, labdanum).

Coffret A gift box containing a selection of miniature bottles of perfume.

Concrete A product obtained in the process of extracting essential oils by volatile solvents. When a waxy substance called stearoptene is removed from this you are left with the absolute (see above). But perfumers often prefer to use the concrete rather than the absolute.

Coniferous note The fragrance of pine, spruce, juniper, and similar trees.

Coumarin A substance found in several plants, and also synthesized from coal tar, which carries the fragrance of new-mown hay.

Distillation The main method of obtaining essential oils from plants, nowadays almost always by using steam rather than boiling water. The oil evaporates and, when condensed back, floats on the surface of the water and is collected. Effectively used by the Arabs from the eighth century AD.

Double scent bottle A perfume bottle popular in mid-Victorian times which opened at both ends, usually with perfume at one end and smelling salts at the other.

Dry perfume A recent development by which tiny, pearlized microcapsules, looking like powder, are placed on the skin and stroked, when they break and release a perfume.

Earthy note A fragrance note giving the impression of earth or earth mold. It is found in certain essential oils like patchouli and vetiver.

Eau de cologne A perfume developed in Cologne in the eighteenth and nineteenth centuries. Nowadays the word signifies a perfume water containing 3–5 percent of perfume oil in a 70 percent alcohol/water mix.

Eau de parfum The strongest mixture of *eau*, usually containing 15–18 percent of perfume oil mixed with an 80–90 percent grade alcohol.

Eau de toilette Also called toilet water. Originally a spirit obtained by distilling fragrant materials in water. Now a standard strength of perfume in which the alcohol contains 4–8 percent perfume.

Eau fraîche A toilet water similar to *eau de cologne* but made with a higher grade of alcohol.

Extraction Also called infusion. The process of obtaining essential oils by dissolving with volatile solvents (such as ether).

Extrait The most concentrated form of perfume sold over the counter. Also called extract and *parfum*. It usually consists of 15–30 percent perfume oil in a high-grade alcohol. A mixture with any lower proportion of perfume oil is called an *eau*.

Factice A very large model of a commercial perfume bottle used for display and advertising.

Fan stopper A fan-shaped perfume-bottle stopper. It may be bigger than the bottle itself.

Fixative Also known as fixator. A perfume ingredient that prolongs the retention of fragrance on the skin and also makes other ingredients in a perfume last longer. Fixatives are mostly gums, resins, and balsams (such as myrrh or galbanum).

Floral perfume A perfume with a fragrance that is predominantly floral.

Floriental An abbreviation for floral-oriental; a perfume containing a balanced mix of floral and oriental notes.

Fougère A fragrance with fresh, herbaceous notes on a mossy, fernlike base. Mostly found in men's fragrances. One of the main perfume categories.

Fragrance blotter Also called smelling strip or *mouillette*. The strip or wand of absorbent paper that perfumers use when testing their fragrances.

Gourmand note Also called edible note. A fragrance evoking a tempting smell of some foodstuff, such as fruit or chocolate.

Green note The general fragrance of grasses and green plant parts in a perfume. Green perfumes form one of the main perfume categories.

Hair powder A perfumed powder much used in the seventeenth and eighteenth centuries for cleaning and smartening wigs.

Herbaceous note The general fragrance of herbs and herbal medicaments.

Hesperidic The fragrance obtained from citrus fruits.

Incense A fragrant smoke produced by burning aromatic substances, often used in religious ceremonies. In early times frankincense was the principal material used, so that in perfumery the words incense and frankincense are now synonymous.

Infusion See *Extraction*

Light notes Notes with a fresh, floral, citrus, fruity, or green content, without sweet or balsamic elements.

Linear fragrance A style of perfume first brought out in the 1980s in which all the notes produce their full effect at the same time and remain constant.

Mossy note The general odor of oils obtained from mosses and lichens.

Neroli An oil steam-distilled from the flowers of the bitter orange tree.

Oriental Also called amber. In perfumery this is a fragrance reminiscent of the East, having a strong exotic spicy or balsamic character. Oriental perfumes form one of the recognized perfume families.

Pomade A perfumed ointment used on the head. Also fat or oil impregnated with essential oil after processing by the enfleurage method. A pomander is a ball of solid, scented material, usually in an ornamental container, carried since ancient times for pleasure or to ward off contagion. Formerly they included ambergris, hence *pomme ambre* (amber apple), from which the name derives.

Potpourri A mixture of fragrant materials, usually dried and including rose petals, placed in a jar or bowl to perfume a room.

Resinoid A resin that has been cleaned by washing with benzene or alcohol.

Sachet A small bag containing dried fragrant materials which is usually laid among clothes or linen to perfume them. Nowadays the word also applies to bags made of plastic and other materials used as a container for liquid.

Sillage (French, pronounced *siyaj*, meaning wake) Also trail. The aroma left by a person wearing perfume who walks past.

Single note A perfume made to provide the scent of a specific flower or a simple posy, with few low notes.

Strewing herb A plant strewn over the floor of a room in medieval times to perfume the air when trodden on.

Sweet note In perfumery this is a sweet, rather sugary fragrance like vanilla.

Synthetic fragrance A laboratory-made imitation of a natural perfume or a fragrance made in a laboratory that does not exist in nature. Many synthetics are derived from natural materials. Geraniol, for example, provides the basic part of the fragrance in a rose, but can be more cheaply and abundantly obtained from a geranium. Several thousand different synthetics are now available for perfumers to use.

Tigella A rod, usually of glass and sometimes sculptured, attached to the underneath of a perfume bottle stopper for use as a dipper.

Toilet water See *Eau de toilette*

Unguent A viscous perfumed ointment, often made by steeping fragrant plants into animal fat, which was used in ancient times.

Vinaigrette A small box with a pierced inner lid containing wool or a sponge which was soaked with aromatic vinegar, for use as a smelling bottle. Vinaigrettes were mostly used in the seventeenth and eighteenth centuries and were usually made of silver and very ornamented.

Washball A perfumed or medicated ball of soap used in the seventeenth and eighteenth centuries when washing the face and hands.

FURTHER READING

Barillé, Elizabeth, and Laroze, Catherine, *The Book of Perfume* (Flammarion, Paris & New York, 1995)

Edwards, Michael, *Perfume Legends—French Feminine Fragrances* (M. Edwards & Company/H.M. Éditions, Levallois, France, 1997)

Groom, Nigel, *The New Perfume Handbook* (Blackie Academic & Professional, London, 1997)

Irvine, Susan, *Perfume: The Creation and Allure of Classic Fragrances* (Aurum, London, 1996)

Jones-North, Jacqueline, *Commercial Perfume Bottles* (Schiffer Publishing, Pennsylvania, 1987)

Kennett, France, *History of Perfume* (Harrap, London, 1975)

Lefkowith, Christie, *The Art of Perfume* (Thames & Hudson, London, 1994)

INDEX

ACKNOWLEDGEMENTS

Bvlgari Parfums: p 36; Chopard: p 12 r; E. T. Archive: pp 8, 9, 10 t, 32 t, 34 r; Floris: p 37 t; The Fragrance
Foundation: pp 32 b, 33, 34 t, bl; Parfums Givenchy: p 12 t; Parfums Lanvin: pp 11 t, 12 c, bl; Estée Lauder: p 10
b; Life File: (Caroline Field) p 17 t; Jo Malone: p 29;
Parfums Rochas: pp 15, 27, 28; Shiseido: p 11 b; Travel Ink: pp 13 (Charcrit Boonsom), 19 b (Charlie Marsden),
20 t (Peter Murphy), 26 (Martyn Hughes).
The publisher would like to thank Mr Lall of Beauty Base Limited (Unit C3, Whiteleys of Bayswater, Queensway,
London W2 4YQ) for supplying a number of perfume bottles for photography.

AUTHOR'S NOTE

So many people have assisted me with information for this book that it is impossible to acknowledge them all by
name. The contribution of each and every one is greatly appreciated. Thanks to my Senior Editor, Clare Hubbard,
who not only kept me on the right track regarding the text but has also diligently looked after the illustrations.